Eating Disorders: Part II

Editors

HARRY A. BRANDT
STEVEN F. CRAWFORD

PSYCHIATRIC CLINICS
OF NORTH AMERICA

www.psych.theclinics.com

Consulting Editor
HARSH K. TRIVEDI

June 2019 • Volume 42 • Number 2

ELSEVIER

1600 John F. Kennedy Boulevard • Suite 1800 • Philadelphia, Pennsylvania, 19103-2899

http://www.theclinics.com

PSYCHIATRIC CLINICS OF NORTH AMERICA Volume 42, Number 2
June 2019 ISSN 0193-953X, ISBN-13: 978-0-323-68213-8

Editor: Lauren Boyle
Developmental Editor: Kristen Helm

Psychiatric Clinics of North America (ISSN 0193-953X) is published quarterly by Elsevier Inc., 360 Park Avenue South, New York, NY 10010-1710. Months of issue are March, June, September, and December. Business and Editorial Offices: 1600 John F. Kennedy Blvd., Suite 1800, Philadelphia, PA 19103-2899. Periodicals postage paid at New York, NY and additional mailing offices. Subscription prices are $332.00 per year (US individuals), $699.00 per year (US institutions), $100.00 per year (US students/residents), $406.00 per year (Canadian individuals), $462.00 per year (international individuals), $880.00 per year (Canadian & international institutions), and $220.00 per year (Canadian & international students/residents). Foreign air speed delivery is included in all *Clinics*' subscription prices. All prices are subject to change without notice. POSTMASTER: Send address changes to *Psychiatric Clinics of North America*, Elsevier Health Sciences Division, Subscription Customer Service, 3251 Riverport Lane, Maryland Heights, MO 63043. **Customer Service: 1-800-654-2452 (US). From outside the United States, call 1-314-447-8871. Fax: 1-314-447-8029. E-mail: journalscustomerservice-usa@elsevier.com (for print support) and journalsonline support-usa@elsevier.com (for online support).**

Reprints. For copies of 100 or more, of articles in this publication, please contact the Commercial Reprints Department, Elsevier Inc., 360 Park Avenue South, New York, New York 10010-1710. Tel.: 212-633-3874, Fax: 212-633-3820, E-mail: reprints@elsevier.com.

Psychiatric Clinics of North America is covered in *MEDLINE/PubMed (Index Medicus)*, *Current Contents/Social and Behavioral Sciences*, *Social Science Citation Index*, *Embase/Excerpta Medica*, and PsycINFO.

Contributors

CONSULTING EDITOR

HARSH K. TRIVEDI, MD, MBA
President & Chief Executive Officer, Sheppard Pratt Health System, Baltimore, Maryland, USA

EDITORS

HARRY A. BRANDT, MD
Co-Director, Center for Eating Disorders at Sheppard Pratt, Chief, Department of Psychiatry, University of Maryland, St. Joseph Medical Center, Clinical Associate Professor, University of Maryland School of Medicine, Towson, Maryland, USA

STEVEN F. CRAWFORD, MD
Co-Director, Center for Eating Disorders at Sheppard Pratt, Assistant Chief, Department of Psychiatry, University of Maryland, St. Joseph Medical Center, Clinical Associate Professor, University of Maryland School of Medicine, Towson, Maryland, USA

AUTHORS

WILLIAM STEWART AGRAS, MD
Professor of Psychiatry (Emeritus), Department of Psychiatry and Behavioral Sciences, Stanford University, Stanford, California, USA

KIMBERLY PEDDICORD ANDERSON, PhD
Director, Department of Psychology, The Center for Eating Disorders at Sheppard Pratt, Baltimore, Maryland, USA

S. BRYN AUSTIN, ScD
Professor, Department of Social and Behavioral Sciences, Harvard T.H. Chan School of Public Health, Professor, Department of Pediatrics, Harvard Medical School, Director of Fellowship Research Training, Division of Adolescent and Young Adult Medicine, Boston Children's Hospital, Director, Strategic Training Initiative for the Prevention of Eating Disorders: A Public Health Incubator, Boston, Massachusetts, USA

CASSIE S. BRODE, PhD
Department of Behavioral Medicine and Psychiatry, West Virginia University School of Medicine, Morgantown, West Virginia, USA

TERRY CARNEY, PhD (Mon), LLB (Hons), Dip Crim (Melb)
Emeritus Professor of Law, School of Law, The University of Sydney, New South Wales, Australia

SCOTT J. CROW, MD
Professor, Department of Psychiatry, University of Minnesota, Minneapolis, Minnesota, USA; The Emily Program, St Paul, Minnesota, USA

ELLEN E. FITZSIMMONS-CRAFT, PhD
Assistant Professor, Department of Psychiatry, Washington University School of Medicine, St Louis, Missouri, USA

JULIE FRIEDMAN, PhD
National Senior Director, Binge Eating Treatment and Recovery, Eating Recovery Center, Assistant Professor, Northwestern University Medical School, Department of Psychiatry, Eating Recovery Center Insight, Chicago, Illinois, USA

DENNIS GIBSON, MD
Assistant Medical Director, ACUTE @ Denver Health, Assistant Professor of Medicine, University of Colorado School of Medicine, Denver, Colorado, USA

SASHA GORRELL, PhD
Postdoctoral Clinical Psychology T32 Scholar, Department of Psychiatry, University of California, San Francisco, San Francisco, California, USA

REBECCA HUTCHESON, MSW
Research Fellow, Strategic Training Initiative for the Prevention of Eating Disorders: A Public Health Incubator, Boston, Massachusetts, USA; Department of Health Services, University of Washington School of Public Health, PhD student, Health and Public Health Systems Research, University of Washington, Seattle, Washington, USA

SARAH JOHNSON, BA
Research Assistant, Oregon Research Institute, Eugene, Oregon, USA

ANNA M. KARAM, MA
Graduate Student, Department of Psychology, Washington University in St. Louis, St Louis, Missouri, USA

DANIEL LE GRANGE, PhD
Benioff UCSF Professor in Children's Health, Director, Eating Disorders Program, Department of Psychiatry, University of California, San Francisco, San Francisco, California, USA; Emeritus Professor of Psychiatry and Behavioral Neuroscience, The University of Chicago, Chicago, Illinois, USA

KATHERINE LOEB, PhD
Professor, School of Psychology, Fairleigh Dickinson University, Teaneck, New Jersey, USA

SARAH MAGUIRE, BSc (Psych) Hons, MA, DCP, PhD
Director, InsideOut Institute, Charles Perkins Centre, University of Sydney, New South Wales, Australia

PHILIP S. MEHLER, MD
President, Eating Recovery Center, Founder and Executive Medical Director, ACUTE @ Denver Health, Glassman Professor of Medicine, University of Colorado School of Medicine, Denver, Colorado, USA

JAMES E. MITCHELL, MD
Department of Psychiatry and Behavioral Science, University of North Dakota School of Medicine and Health Sciences, Grand Forks, North Dakota, USA

CAROL B. PETERSON, PhD
Associate Professor, Department of Psychiatry, University of Minnesota, Minneapolis, Minnesota, USA

EMILY M. PISETSKY, PhD
Assistant Professor, Department of Psychiatry, University of Minnesota, Minneapolis, Minnesota, USA

BRONWYN RAYKOS, PhD
Centre for Clinical Interventions, Northbridge, Australia

LAUREN M. SCHAEFER, PhD
Postdoctoral Fellow, Sanford Center for Biobehavioral Research, Fargo, North Dakota, USA

ULRIKE SCHMIDT, MD, PhD, FRCPsych
Head of the Department of Psychological Medicine, Professor, Section of Eating Disorders, King's College London, Institute of Psychiatry, Psychology and Neuroscience, The Eating Disorders Service, Maudsley Hospital, Consultant Psychiatrist, South London and Maudsley NHS Foundation Trust, London, United Kingdom

LAURA ELIZABETH SPROCH, PhD
Research Coordinator, Department of Psychology, The Center for Eating Disorders at Sheppard Pratt, Baltimore, Maryland, USA

ERIC STICE, PhD
Senior Scientist, Oregon Research Institute, Eugene, Oregon, USA

MARIAN TANOFSKY-KRAFF, PhD
Professor, Department of Medical and Clinical Psychology, Uniformed Services University of the Health Sciences (USUHS), Bethesda, Maryland, USA

STEPHEN WILLIAM TOUYZ, BSc (Cape Town), BSc (Hons) (Wits), PhD (Cape Town)
Professor of Clinical Psychology, School of Psychology and Inside Out Institute, University of Sydney, Brain Mind Centre, Camperdown, New South Wales, Australia

ROXANE TURGON, MA
PhD Student, University Grenoble Alpes, LIP/PC2, Universite Grenoble Alpes, Grenoble, France

KATRINA VELASQUEZ, Esq, MA
Managing Principal, Center Road Solutions, LLC, Washington, DC, USA

GLENN WALLER, DPhil
Department of Psychology, University of Sheffield, Sheffield, United Kingdom

ELIZABETH WASSENAAR, MS, MD
Associate Medical Director, Eating Recovery Center, Denver, Colorado, USA

SHALINI WICKRAMATILAKE-TEMPLEMAN, MHS
Visiting Scholar, Strategic Training Initiative for the Prevention of Eating Disorders: A Public Health Incubator, Boston, Massachusetts, USA

DENISE E. WILFLEY, PhD
Scott Rudolph University, Professor of Psychiatry, Medicine, Pediatrics, and Psychological and Brain Sciences, Washington University School of Medicine, St Louis, Missouri, USA

STEPHEN A. WONDERLICH, PhD
President and Scientific Director, Sanford Center for Biobehavioral Research, Fargo, North Dakota, USA; Chester Fritz Distinguished Professor, University of North Dakota School of Medicine and Health Sciences, Grand Forks, North Dakota, USA

CASSANDRA WORKMAN, MD
Eating Recovery Center, Denver, Colorado, USA

JOEL YAGER, MD
Professor, Department of Psychiatry, University of Colorado School of Medicine, Aurora, Colorado, USA

SEE HENG YIM, BSc
Research Assistant, Section of Eating Disorders, King's College London, Institute of Psychiatry, Psychology and Neuroscience, London, United Kingdom

Contents

Selected Treatments for Eating Disorders

Cognitive behavioral therapy (CBT) is an evidence-based treatment for bulimia nervosa and binge-eating disorder and is regarded as the first-line treatment for both eating disorders. An enhanced version of the treatment (CBT-E) appears more effective in treating patients with severe comorbidity. There is less evidence that CBT is effective for the treatment of anorexia nervosa. Evidence suggests that CBT-E is no more effective than specialist care involving regular medical follow-up and supportive psychotherapy in the persistent adult form of anorexia nervosa (AN). Early studies suggest that CBT-E may be useful in treating the adolescent form of AN.

Behavioral methods are inherent in many evidence-based treatments of eating disorders and have also been used separately. This review demonstrates that behavioral methods are necessary in the effective treatment of eating disorders—in particular, the improvement of nutrition and exposure-based methods. It is also possible that these methods are sufficient to treat anorexia nervosa, although other elements are needed on the treatment of bulimia nervosa. The impacts and mechanisms of behavioral and nutritional change merit serious attention in clinical work and research. Clinicians are often reluctant, however, to use these methods, and that needs to be the focus of supervision.

Eating disorders (EDs) are serious psychiatric illnesses that typically develop during adolescence or young adulthood, indicating that individuals with EDs may benefit from early intervention. Family-based treatment is the leading treatment of youth with anorexia nervosa, with increasing evidence of its efficacy for youth with bulimia nervosa. This review describes the role of family engagement within family-based treatment of EDs, followed by a summary of current empirically supported, family-based ED interventions. It concludes with discussion of the ways in which family interventions are expanding and adapting to improve the breadth and scope of ED treatment in adolescence and young adulthood.

Interpersonal psychotherapy (IPT) for the treatment of eating disorders is a brief treatment that addresses the social and interpersonal context in which the disorder begins and is maintained. IPT is classified as a strongly supported evidence-based treatment of bulimia nervosa and binge-eating disorder, and more research is needed to understand the effectiveness of IPT for anorexia nervosa and IPT for preventing excess weight gain. This article describes the core components and elements of IPT, the empirical evidence that supports its effectiveness, efforts to increase the dissemination and implementation of IPT, and future directions.

The authors present the theoretic model, structure of treatment, and preliminary evidence for several emerging treatments that are increasingly being used and studied in eating disorders treatment, including dialectical behavior therapy, acceptance and commitment therapy, integrative cognitive-affective therapy, and neuromodulation. In addition, the article discusses treatments that address mindfulness, interpersonal factors, and habit.

The authors provide an overview of the current state of research on self-help interventions for eating disorders. The efficacy of different forms of self-help interventions for bulimia nervosa, binge eating disorder, and other eating disorders at various stages of the care pathway (from prevention to relapse prevention) is described. Cost-effectiveness studies are also presented. Moderators of outcome, such as guidance and adherence, are discussed. Overall, the findings are promising and support the use of self-help interventions in the treatment of bulimic disorders, across the stages of the care pathway. Less is known about the use of self-help in anorexia nervosa.

The delivery of teletherapy is an important advancement in clinical care for the treatment of eating disorders (EDs). Specifically, it seems to improve access to highly specialized ED treatment. Research on the application of videoconferencing-based psychotherapy services for EDs is minimal; however, results suggest that this treatment format leads to significant improvements in clinical symptoms and is well accepted by patients. General telemedicine guidelines and administrative and clinical recommendations specific to the treatment of ED patients have been identified. With careful planning and thoughtful application, Internet-based therapy seems to be a valuable resource for practitioners seeking to disseminate specialized ED treatments.

Scott J. Crow

Medications are a useful adjunct to nutritional and psychotherapeutic treatments for eating disorders. Antidepressants are commonly used to treat bulimia nervosa; high-dose fluoxetine is a standard approach, but many other antidepressants can be used. Binge eating disorder can be treated with antidepressants, with medications that diminish appetite, or with lisdexamfetamine. Anorexia nervosa does not generally respond to medications, although recent evidence supports modest weight restoration benefits from olanzapine.

Medical Complications of Eating Disorders

Dennis Gibson, Cassandra Workman, and Philip S. Mehler

Anorexia nervosa and bulimia nervosa are mental illnesses with associated complications affecting all body systems with arguably the highest mortality of all mental health disorders. A comprehensive medical evaluation is an essential first step in the treatment of anorexia nervosa and bulimia nervosa. Weight restoration and cessation of purging behaviors are often essential components in the management of medical complications of these illnesses.

Elizabeth Wassenaar, Julie Friedman, and Philip S. Mehler

Binge eating disorder (BED) is the most common eating disorder and is accompanied by multiple medical comorbidities, many of which are associated with obesity-related diseases. However, the BED itself is likely to confer additional risk factors. BED presents with medical symptoms in virtually every body system and can have devastating consequences on both quality and length of life. This review covers the major comorbidities of BED and highlights areas of ongoing research in this disorder.

Special Topics

Cassie S. Brode and James E. Mitchell

Bariatric surgery candidates often report problematic and/or eating disordered behaviors. For most patients, these eating behaviors improve after surgery. A subset, however, experience a recurrence or new onset of problematic eating behaviors as early as 2 months to 18 months after surgery, which can result in compromised weight loss/excessive weight regain. Those most at risk are individuals with comorbid psychopathology (ie, loss-of-control eating or depression) after surgery. For some, such problems are present before surgery. Therefore, it is critical to monitor patients closely after surgery so that appropriate psychiatric treatments can be provided if indicated.

The issues centering on the involuntary treatment of severe and enduring anorexia nervosa are daunting. There is a general consensus that people with this illness are likely to have high levels of disability, be underemployed/unemployed, and receive welfare. Anorexia nervosa shows a similar degree of impairment to those with depression or schizophrenia on quality-of-life measures. It is possible to mount a cogent argument as to why a rehabilitation model of care needs to be considered for those with persistent eating disorders. In such cases, harm minimization and improved quality of life should be prioritized and involuntary treatment used judiciously.

Thirteen percent of girls and women experience an eating disorder, yet most do not receive treatment. Thus, broad implementation of eating disorder prevention programs that reduce eating disorder symptoms and future eating disorder onset is a critical priority. This article (1) reviews risk factors that have been shown to predict future onset of eating disorders, because this should guide the content of prevention programs and high-risk subgroups to target with selective prevention programs; (2) reviews the evidence base for eating disorder prevention programs that have reduced eating disorder symptoms or future onset of eating disorders; and (3) discusses directions for future research.

Over the past decade, a first wave of US public policy advocacy for eating disorders made substantial progress, with passage of the federal 21st Century Cures Act in 2016 as its crowning achievement. However, the US response to eating disorders continues to fall short in several ways. On the cusp of a second wave of policy advocacy, efforts must be broadened to target structural determinants of illness and inequities to maximize clinical impact and diminish suffering. Mental health clinicians, patients, and their families will be essential players in public policy advocacy efforts in this regard.

PSYCHIATRIC CLINICS OF NORTH AMERICA

FORTHCOMING ISSUES

September 2019
Professional Development for Psychiatrists
Howard Y. Liu and Donald Hilty, *Editors*

December 2019
Integrating Technology into 21st Century Psychiatry: Telemedicine, Social Media, and other Technologies
James H. Shore, *Editor*

March 2020
Mixed Affective States: Beyond Current Boundaries
Alan C. Swann and Gabriele Sani, *Editors*

RECENT ISSUES

March 2019
Eating Disorders: Part I
Harry A. Brandt and Steven F. Crawford, *Editors*

December 2018
Borderline Personality Disorder
Frank Yeomans and Kenneth N. Levy, *Editors*

September 2018
Neuromodulation
Scott T. Aaronson and Noah S. Philip, *Editors*

SERIES OF RELATED INTEREST

Child and Adolescent Psychiatric Clinics of North America
Neurologic Clinics

Preface

New Developments in the Clinical Treatment of Eating Disorders

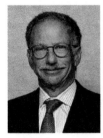
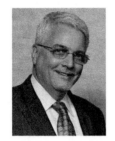

Harry A. Brandt, MD   Steven F. Crawford, MD
Editors

The eating disorders, because of their etiologic complexity and significant morbidity and mortality, often wreak havoc on patients and their families and pose vexing clinical challenges to treating clinicians. We were so very pleased that the *Psychiatric Clinics of North America* recognized the critical need for a comprehensive update on these serious illnesses and asked us to gather a group of the most renowned and distinguished international leaders in our field to collaborate in providing it. In part 1, we address the core issues in the diagnosis and classification of the major eating disorders as well as review some of the many progress areas in current clinical research. Using this as a foundation, part 2 provides a review of the most up-to-date evidence-based treatment strategies.

Part 2 begins with an overview of selected treatments for eating disorders. Cognitive behavioral therapy (CBT) is reviewed by our friend and long-time collaborator, Dr Stewart Agras. CBT stands out as perhaps the most studied and evidence-based treatment for bulimia nervosa (BN) and binge-eating disorder (BED). Drs Glenn Waller and Bronwyn Raykos follow with further discussion of behavioral intervention for eating disorders promoting nutritional change through exposure and skills development. Drs Sasha Gorrell, Katherine Loeb, and Daniel Le Grange then provide a compelling review and update on family-based treatments, considered by many to be the treatment of choice for adolescents with anorexia nervosa. Anna Karam, MA and Drs Ellen

Psychiatr Clin N Am 42 (2019) xiii–xv
https://doi.org/10.1016/j.psc.2019.03.001
0193-953X/19/© 2019 Published by Elsevier Inc.

psych.theclinics.com

Fitzsimmons-Craft, Marian Tanofsky-Kraff, and Denise Wilfley review the use of interpersonal psychotherapy for eating disorders. This is followed by a discussion of other emerging innovations in psychological treatments, including dialectical behavioral therapy, acceptance and commitment therapy, integrative cognitive-affective therapy, and neuromodulation by Drs Emily Pisetsky, Lauren Schaefer, Stephen Wonderlich, and Carol Peterson. See Heng Yim and Dr Ulrike Schmidt review our current understanding of the efficacy of self-help interventions for BN and BED, highlighting important areas for future research. Drs Laura Sproch and Kimberly Anderson from our center then present a review of the use of clinician-delivered teletherapies for eating disorders, which we hope will encourage wider dissemination of important treatments to outlying areas. Dr Scott Crow completes this section of the issue by providing a comprehensive and thoughtful review of the current recommendations regarding pharmacologic treatments.

The second section of the issue provides a review of medical complications associated with eating disorders. First, Drs Dennis Gibson, Cassandra Workman, and Philip Mehler provide an update on the medical complications and their treatments for anorexia nervosa and BN; this is followed by review of the same for BED by Drs Elizabeth Wassenaar, Julie Friedman, and Philip Mehler.

The final section of the issue explores other topics that we felt were timely and important in completing a comprehensive overview of eating disorders. Drs Cassie Brode and James Mitchell lead by addressing problematic eating behaviors and eating disorders associated with bariatric surgery, an important area in light of the increasing use of this intervention. This is followed by a review of the complexities seen in the involuntary treatment of patients with eating disorders authored by Drs Terry Carney, Joel Yager, Sarah Maguire, and Stephen Touyz. Next, Dr Eric Stice, Sarah Johnson, BA, and Roxane Turgon, MA present an overview on the current thinking on eating disorder prevention. Part 2 then concludes with a thorough discussion of the second wave of public policy advocacy for eating disorders by S. Bryn Austin, ScD, Rebecca Hutcheson, MSW, Shalini Wickramatilake-Templeman, MHS, and Katrina Velasquez, Esq, MA.

It is our sincere hope that this update on eating disorders will be of utility to a wide range of primary clinicians as well as specialists as they attempt to find their way in helping individuals with eating disorders and their families. On a personal note, we offer our sincere thanks to Dr Harsh Trivedi for inviting us to edit these issues, as well as the staff at Elsevier, who made this daunting task a bit more manageable by providing useful counsel and structure and many gentle pushes to keep us on task. Most of all, we are grateful to the authors, many of whom are our close friends with whom we have collaborated for decades. We appreciate their gracious willingness to embark on this project with us.

Harry A. Brandt, MD
Center for Eating Disorders at
Sheppard Pratt
Department of Psychiatry
University of Maryland
St. Joseph Medical Center
Physician Pavilion North, Suite 300
6535 North Charles Street
Towson, MD 21204, USA

Steven F. Crawford, MD
Center for Eating Disorders at
Sheppard Pratt
University of Maryland
St. Joseph Medical Center
Physician Pavilion North, Suite 300
6535 North Charles Street
Towson, MD 21204, USA

E-mail addresses:
harry@brandtmd.com (H.A. Brandt)
scrawford@sheppardpratt.org (S.F. Crawford)

Selected Treatments for Eating Disorders

Cognitive Behavior Therapy for the Eating Disorders

William Stewart Agras, MD

KEYWORDS

- Cognitive behavioral therapy • Anorexia nervosa • Bulimia nervosa
- Binge eating disorder • CBT • CBT-E

KEY POINTS

- Cognitive behavior therapy (CBT) is an evidence-based treatment for bulimia nervosa and binge-eating disorder.
- The briefer guided self-help form of CBT is effective in the treatment of binge-eating disorder and may be used as a first step in the treatment of bulimia nervosa.
- CBT-E (broad form) is likely more effective in patients with eating disorder with more severe comorbidity.
- The role of CBT is uncertain in the treatment of both adult and adolescent anorexia nervosa.

OVERVIEW

Cognitive-behavioral therapy (CBT) is an evidence-based treatment for bulimia nervosa (BN) and binge-eating disorder (BED), and may be useful in the treatment of anorexia nervosa (AN).[1,2] Most treatment guidelines consider CBT to be the first-line treatment for BN and BED.[3] Clinical observations led to a greater understanding of the influences maintaining BN and to an enhanced version of CBT (CBT-E).[1,4] At the same time, a transdiagnostic view of eating disorders was developed, noting that the core psychopathology was similar in all the eating disorders, with the adapted CBT-E regarded as a treatment for all eating disorders.[5] Four additional processes were theorized to maintain eating disorders in CBT-E. The first is extreme perfectionism.[6] The second involves faulty coping with intense mood states, including depression, anxiety, and anger.[6] The third is low core self-esteem, and the fourth interpersonal difficulties. For patients who are not progressing well, an evaluation of the potential role of each of these processes in maintaining the illness is of prime importance.

The effectiveness of CBT for the treatment of eating disorders has been confirmed in a number of clinical trials.[7–14] Overall, CBT has been found as, or more effective, than

Disclosure Statement: The author have no conflict of interest in writing this article.
Department of Psychiatry and Behavioral Sciences, Stanford University, 401 Quarry Road, #1322, Stanford, CA 94305, USA
E-mail address: sagras@stanford.edu

Psychiatr Clin N Am 42 (2019) 169–179
https://doi.org/10.1016/j.psc.2019.01.001
0193-953X/19/© 2019 Elsevier Inc. All rights reserved.

other treatment approaches, such as medication and other psychotherapies for eating disorders, except for AN.[15,16]

COGNITIVE BEHAVIOR THERAPY MODEL

BN develops in the context of weight loss consequent on dieting driven by concerns about body shape and weight. Dieting that produces a caloric deficit eventually leads to binge eating, and in patients with BN to compensatory behaviors such as self-induced vomiting, diuretic and laxative abuse, and excessive exercise. Binge eating is associated with a sense of loss of control over eating and is characterized by excessive caloric intake. Repeated failures to avoid binge eating and purging result in a negative mood and low self-esteem. This, in turn, reinforces weight and shape concerns continuing the inexorable cycle of dieting, binge eating, and purging.

COGNITIVE BEHAVIOR THERAPY

As shown in **Fig. 1**, there are several areas that could form a focus for intervention. However, in the first third of treatment with CBT, the primary aim is to reduce dietary restriction. The first step is to create an agreed formulation of the factors maintaining the disorder with the patient (**Box 1**). This is achieved using the CBT model (see **Fig. 1**) as a basis for education and discussion. Weekly weighing with the therapist is instituted from the first session and continues throughout treatment. Even though patients often want to weigh more often they are discouraged from doing so, pointing out that daily weight fluctuations that have no physiologic meaning only add to worry about body weight and shape.

Self-monitoring of dietary intake, binge eating, and purging and the circumstances in which they occur provide data for both the therapist and patient. An example of self-monitoring from a patient with BN is shown in **Table 1**. As can be seen, the patient eats very little between 9 AM and 12:15 PM, leaving her hungry and anxious as she looks forward to lunch with her boyfriend. She then sets herself up for a binge by allowing herself to loosen control over her eating when she decided that she was going to purge. The binge was then followed by vomiting and taking 2 diuretics. Shortly afterward, she ate a piece of chocolate and purged again "wanting an empty

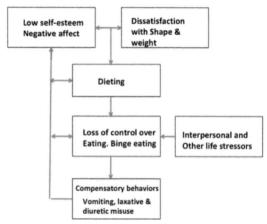

Fig. 1. Cognitive-behavioral model of factors influencing the development of eating disorders.

Box 1
Elements of cognitive-behavioral therapy

Phase 1

- Patient/Therapist agree on factors influencing the eating disorder
- Weekly weighing with therapist
- Self-monitoring
- Eating by the clock

Phase 2

- Review of progress
- Adjust focus of treatment if needed

Phase 3

- Introduction of feared foods
- Address weight and shape concerns
- Address triggers of binge eating; for example, interpersonal conflicts

Phase 4

- Review of progress in reducing factors influencing the eating disorder
- Consider future triggers for relapse
- Discuss strategies in reducing risk

Those interested in online training in enhanced cognitive behavior therapy should contact Marianne.oconnor@psych.ox.as.uk.

stomach." An evening binge occurred at home followed by episodes of vomiting. She ends the day with 2 diuretics.

Self-monitoring provides the data allowing recognition of the restricted eating patterns as a basis for instituting a regular pattern of eating by the clock consisting of 3 meals and 2 snacks each day adjusted to the patient's lifestyle. In the case illustrated in **Table 1**, the first aim would be to increase food intake at breakfast and follow this with a snack at approximately 10:30 AM, lunch at 12:30 PM, a snack at 3:30 PM, and dinner at 6:30 PM. Another snack may be needed before bedtime. Regular eating reduces the intervals between eating episodes, thus reducing hunger, loss of control, binge eating, and therefore purging. Studies have shown that increased regularity of eating is associated with symptom reduction and with abstinence from, or reduction of binge eating/purging[17–19]; hence, the frequency of purging should begin to decrease as regular eating is established. Education about the futility of using laxatives and diuretics because they result in dehydration and not fat loss is useful at this point. Depending on the situation, these forms of purging can be slowly phased out or in some cases simply stopped.

Studies have shown that if purging is reduced by 60% at session 4 of treatment, the chance of a favorable outcome is greater than for those who fail to reach this criterion.[20–22] This measure provides an opportunity for patient and therapist to review progress early in treatment, to discuss reasons why progress is slow, and to adjust the therapeutic focus. At this point, triggers of binge eating should be explored through the data collected in self-monitoring and solutions to these issues addressed through formal problem solving.

As eating becomes more regular, the focus of treatment shifts to the content of food with the aim of increasing the variety of foods consumed and slowly introducing

Table 1
Example of a self-monitoring form filled out for 1 day by a patient with bulimia nervosa

Time	Food Intake	Location	Binge	Purge	Situation
9.00 AM	³/₄ red apple			2 D	Woke up feeling bloated
12.15–1.15 PM	Chinese chicken salad 1 small plate. Chicken with water chestnuts ½ cup 5 honey walnut shrimp 4 Szechuan shrimp Chow mein 1/3 cup Chicken & vegetable sauce 1 cup Steamed rice 1 cup 2 diet cokes, 1 cup tea, water	HoChow restaurant with boy friend	B	V 2D	Before lunch hungry and anxious. Overwhelmed when food came; after first bites I decided I was going to purge, ate more than I wanted
1:30 PM	1 piece of chocolate, water	At work		V	Felt ashamed of binge and wanted an empty stomach
4:15 PM	24 oz diet coke	At work			Started to feel hungry
5:40 PM	4 Szechuan shrimp	In car	B		Leftovers from lunch
7:00 PM	1/3 cup chicken and water chestnuts 1 cheese enchilada 2 cups leftover Chinese food 2 large chocolate chip cookies	In kitchen	B		Wanting powdered sugar covered donuts, frantic feeling, mad with myself
7:45 PM	1 peanut cluster, 6 Oreo cookies	Lucky's in car		V	
8:10 PM	1 pint B&J ice cream, chocolate fudge brownie	Bedroom		V	
10:30 PM				2 D	

Abbreviation: B, binge; D, diuretic; V, vomiting.

avoided foods beginning with foods that cause the least anxiety. The aim here is to decrease dietary restraint by widening the range of food choices.

When regular eating is established with a continuing reduction of binge eating and purging, the focus shifts to the overvaluation of shape and weight. The consequences of overvaluation are discussed and elaborated with the patient and attention given to reducing the amount of body checking. Avoidance of activities based on body dissatisfaction also should be explored and homework developed to overcome such avoidance. The final sessions focus on maintenance of the progress made, how to deal with lapses, and taking a realistic view of the future. The usual length of treatment is 18 to 20 sessions.

APPLICATIONS TO CLINICAL SYNDROMES
Bulimia Nervosa

The existing clinical trials indicate that CBT is superior to wait-list controls, placebo conditions, and other psychotherapies such as interpersonal psychotherapy (IPT) and psychodynamic psychotherapy (PDT). Two recent meta-analyses came to similar conclusions.[23,24] The first, a network analysis that allows comparisons of all treatments to each other, found that CBT was likely the most effective treatment for BN. The second meta-analysis came to a similar, but slightly stronger conclusion that therapist-led CBT was more effective than wait-list conditions, interpersonal and other psychotherapies to which it has been compared.

However, differences between CBT and IPT tend to disappear during follow-up. For example, in a trial comparing CBT and IPT for BN, CBT was significantly superior to IPT in the proportions of patients recovered and remitted at end of treatment[8]; however, at follow-up, there was no significant difference between groups. It seems that IPT, perhaps because the focus of treatment is not directly on the eating-disordered behaviors of BN but rather on interpersonal behaviors, works more slowly. In the second study, CBT-E was found superior to IPT at posttreatment for the primary outcome, percent remitted (CBT 65.5%; IPT 33.3%) and at 12-month follow-up (CBT-E 69.4%; IPT 49.0%).[9] The finding that IPT has a slower effect on eating-disordered symptoms than CBT was replicated in this study. It is reasonable to conclude from these findings that IPT is a reliable second-line treatment for BN and may be particularly useful in patients with marked interpersonal issues that trigger binge eating.

An important question is whether CBT is as, or more effective than psychodynamic psychotherapy given that many practicing psychotherapists use the latter treatment. Two randomized controlled trials comparing CBT-E and psychodynamic psychotherapy came to different conclusions on this question.[25,26] In the first study,[25] 70 patients with BN were randomized to 20 sessions of CBT-E or the focused form of psychoanalytic psychotherapy in weekly sessions over a period of 2 years. The results were dramatically in favor of CBT-E both after 20 weeks (CBT-E 42% abstinent; psychoanalytic psychotherapy 6%) and at the 2-year assessment (CBT-E 44% abstinent; psychoanalytic psychotherapy 15%). It is important to note that this study was carried out at a site that had developed the psychoanalytic psychotherapy and that therapists from that site were trained in CBT-E. The second study randomized 81 women with BN or partial BN to up to 60 sessions of either CBT or PDT over a 12-month period. It should be noted that this is far more than the usual number of sessions for CBT, and that the primary outcome was not meeting diagnostic criteria for BN (full or partial), a less stringent definition of remission. For CBT, 33.3% and for PDT, 31.0% no longer met criteria for BN with similar results at 12-month follow-up. However, the effect sizes for reductions in binge eating and purging favored CBT. It is difficult to compare the 2 studies because of differences in those entered to the study, different lengths of treatment, and a different definition of outcome. However, even in the second study, CBT was more effective in reducing binge eating and purging. Hence, the evidence suggests that CBT is more cost-effective because fewer sessions are needed and more effective in reducing binge eating/purging.

Guided self-help

A brief form of CBT has been found effective in reducing binge eating and purging in a number of clinical trials.[27,28] Treatment sessions are usually shorter than in full CBT, for example, 30 minutes, and fewer in number, for example, 8 to 10, with less experienced therapists. Books for the lay population, such as Fairburn's *Overcoming Binge Eating*,[29] are often used, with the therapist supporting the patient in making the needed behavior changes. Hence, the patient becomes responsible for behavior change with the therapist acting as a coach. Guided self-help (GSH) has been shown to be more effective than no treatment, and in some studies as effective as full CBT.[11]

However, the overall effect size of treatment is small, leading to the recommendation that GSH may be best used as a first step in the treatment of BN with a step-up to full CBT if necessary. The fact that GSH is based on the principles of CBT makes step-up to full CBT relatively easy.

Is enhanced cognitive behavior therapy more effective than cognitive behavior therapy?

This question is not easy to answer because there have been few studies that have compared CBT-E with CBT. One relevant study compared the focused form of CBT (a revised form of CBT) with the broad form of CBT-E for individuals with BN and borderline personality disorder.[30] This subgroup of individuals tends to have a worse outcome with treatment than individuals without borderline personality disorder and the associated behavioral and affective symptoms. Fifty women meeting criteria for BN were randomly allocated to the 2 treatments. At the end of treatment and all follow-up points there was no difference in outcome between the 2 treatments, with 42% of individuals achieving remission. However, a moderator analysis found that participants with more severe affective and interpersonal psychopathology had better outcomes with CBT-E. Hence, it seems likely that CBT-E with the extra modules is more effective for individuals with severe comorbid psychopathology.

Applications to adolescents

Relatively few studies are available for CBT applied to adolescents with BN. An uncontrolled study of 68 adolescents with an eating disorder who were not under-weight (approximately 30% BN) and treated with 20 sessions of CBT-E found that half had stopped binge eating/purging at the end of treatment, suggesting that the outcome for adolescents with BN is similar to that of adults. The adolescents' parents were involved at a baseline session and for 4 brief sessions during the course of treatment. The first controlled study compared CBT guided self-help (CBTgsh) with family therapy adapted for BN,[31] finding that CBTgsh was superior to family therapy at the end of treatment, but that at 6-month follow-up there were no differences between treatments, with approximately 55% of adolescents remitted in both groups at that point. Another study compared CBT with family-based treatment (FBT),[32] entering 130 adolescent participants with BN to the study. FBT was superior to CBT both at the end of treatment and at 6-month follow-up, but not at 12-month follow-up when 49% of the FBT group was remitted compared with 32% of the CBT group. Given these different outcomes, it would seem that both CBT and FBT are reasonable treatments for adolescents with BN. However, CBTgsh is less costly to provide and on those grounds may be the preferred treatment, although further studies in adolescents are needed before firm conclusions as to relative efficacy can be drawn.

Binge-Eating Disorder

BED is characterized by episodes of loss of control over eating accompanied by binge eating with no compensatory behaviors. Binges are smaller than in BN probably because no calories are lost by means of self-induced vomiting. Comorbid psychopathology is as frequent and as severe as in BN. In the clinic setting, most patients with BED are overweight or obese, although BED is not necessarily related to being overweight. Because of the similarity between BN and BED, the therapeutic model is identical and CBT can be applied without modification. However, because many patients wish to lose weight, it is necessary to ensure that they do not engage in restricted eating but rather gradually adopt a healthy diet that can be sustained over time. Recovery rates tend to be higher in BED than in BN, perhaps because the placebo response is larger in BED.[33]

The difference in short-term outcomes favoring CBT over IPT in BN does not replicate in BED, in which the 2 treatments appear similar both in short-term and long-term outcome.[12,13] A recent meta-analysis suggested that CBT was superior to behavioral weight-loss treatment (BWL) in short-term follow-up in reducing binge eating.[34] In a study with a 2-year follow-up, 208 individuals were randomly allocated to 1 of 3 groups: CBTgsh, BWL, and IPT.[14] At the end of treatment there was no difference among the 3 groups in reducing binge eating, although BWL was more effective in reducing weight at this point. At the 2-year follow-up there was no difference between groups in weight loss. However, both CBTgsh and IPT were superior to BWL in reducing binge eating with no difference between these 2 treatments. Hence, full CBT, CBTgsh, or IPT seem useful as first-line treatments for BED.

Enhancing cognitive behavior therapy

CBT results in remission or significant improvement in symptoms in approximately 50% to 60% of patients with BN and BED. Hence, the question arises whether adding medication or another psychotherapy might enhance the results of CBT. Several controlled studies have examined the addition of medication to CBT.[16] The most common medication has been an antidepressant such as imipramine, desipramine, or fluoxetine.[7] None of these additions was more effective than CBT alone in reducing binge eating or purging, although one study reported a significant lowering of depression over that produced by CBT alone. Hence, there is no evidence that antidepressants enhance the effectiveness of CBT in reducing binge eating or purging. Even fewer studies have examined the utility of adding another psychotherapy to enhance CBT. The addition of interpersonal psychotherapy for those not responding to CBT did not enhance outcome in a study that added IPT to those who failed to respond well to CBT.[35] Hence, apart from CBT-E probably adding to the effectiveness of CBT in patients with severe comorbidities, no other psychotherapy enhances reductions of binge eating and purging.

Anorexia Nervosa

In considering treatments for AN, it is necessary to take into account 2 different phases of the disorder: the acute phase in adolescence and the persistent phase usually evident in adults. Persistent AN is a chronic disorder characterized by low weight and physiologic instability, accompanied by comorbid psychopathology, particularly depression, obsessive-compulsive and other anxiety disorders, social disability, and one of the highest rates of death for any psychiatric disorder. Deaths are due to either medical complications of chronic starvation or to suicide. The clinical picture is often further complicated by the patient's refusal to cooperate with treatment. The relative rarity of the disorder adds difficulty to the recruitment of adequate sample sizes for controlled studies of treatment modalities, resulting in some uncertainty in considering the relative efficacy of different treatment approaches. Hence, sample sizes are often small and dropout rates are high, making it difficult to draw certain conclusions about relative efficacy.[36,37]

The treatment of the adolescent form of the disorder is somewhat easier because despite the resistance to treatment shown by many adolescents, the family is a valuable resource to manage and stabilize the situation. Hence, treatment dropout rates tend to be lower in adolescents than in adults. The most researched treatment is FBT that results in some 40% of patients remitted and more than

60% improved and hence has become recommended as a first-line treatment for adolescent AN.

Cognitive behavior therapy–enhanced

The enhanced form of CBT is based on a similar model to the other eating disorders with concerns about weight and shape driving dieting, leading to weight loss and maintenance of those losses.[1,4] However, approximately half the patients lose control over their dietary restriction and begin to binge eat and to use compensatory behaviors such as self-induced vomiting, laxative misuse, and overexercise. In the first phase of treatment, the focus is on helping the patient to understand the factors maintaining the disorder. This is followed by a detailed examination of the motivation to continue dieting and weight loss so that patients better understands their eating disorder. The evidence for and against changing their eating behavior is then examined and if the patient is willing to continue treatment, the focus becomes weight gain with gradual modification of the patient's dietary intake using self-monitoring and weekly weighing by the therapist before the treatment session. The reason for the therapist to do the weighing is that the patient's concerns about weight are often provoked by weighing and can be dealt with either immediately or in the session. Concerns about weight and shape are addressed in detail, as are perfectionism, intense mood states, and interpersonal problems. Up to 40 treatment sessions are recommended for AN. The treatment adapted for adolescents includes brief sessions with the parents. In these sessions, factors within the family that may be maintaining the disorder and barriers to treatment are explored. However, the main focus is on dietary advice and the conduct of family meals.

Two meta-analyses considering treatment for persistent AN came to similar conclusions, that in comparing treatment approaches, no one treatment was more effective than another.[36,37] Hence, CBT was no more effective than other psychotherapies with which it was compared. In one multicenter controlled trial, 120 individuals meeting criteria for AN were randomized to 3 treatments: CBT-E, Maudsley Anorexia Nervosa Treatment (MANTRA), and specialist supportive clinical management (SSCM).[38] MANTRA is accompanied by a workbook and is individually tailored to each patient. The foci of treatment include the patient's thinking and relational style, family members responses to the illness, and beliefs about the usefulness of AN in the patient's life. SSCM consisted of clinical management together with supportive psychotherapy focused on normalization of eating and weight restoration. Forty percent of patients did not complete treatment, which did not differ among groups. Patients showed similar improvement in all 3 groups, with approximately 50% of the remaining patients achieving a healthy weight (body mass index >18.5) that was largely maintained at the 1-year follow-up.

Applications to adolescents

There are relatively few studies applying CBT to adolescents with AN. A meta-analysis that separated adolescent and adult studies found that for adolescents, FBT was more effective than individual psychotherapy; however, there were too few comparisons to ensure firm conclusions.[39] At this point, there have been no controlled comparisons of FBT and CBT-E. In one cohort study, 46 patients were treated with CBT-E.[40] The treatment was similar to that for adults except that parents were seen during the 40-session course of therapy. The dropout rate was 40%. At the end of treatment, 22% of patients were remitted with their weight at or above 95% of their expected weight in the intent-to-treat cohort. During a 1-year follow-up, the proportion of remitted patients increased to 28%.

SUMMARY

Most patients with an eating disorder, whether adolescents or adults, can be treated on an outpatient basis. CBT is an effective, evidence-based, first-line treatment for BN and BED. The enhanced form of the treatment is probably more effective in treating patients with severe comorbid psychopathology than the original form of the treatment. The GSH form of CBT can be applied by less specialized therapists and hence may be useful in situations in which there are no therapists able to administer CBT. In addition, many experts recommend that CBTgsh be used as a first step in the treatment of BN and particularly for BED, in which it has been shown to have short-term and long-term effects comparable to other evidence-based treatments. The choice of psychotherapy for the persistent form of AN is more difficult in that no specialized psychotherapy, including CBT-E, has been shown to be more effective than specialized clinical management. There is only preliminary evidence of the effectiveness of CBT-E in the treatment of the adolescent form of AN, and a specific form of FBT is likely the most effective approach to adolescent AN.

REFERENCES

1. Fairburn CG, Cooper Z, Shafran R. Enhanced cognitive behavior therapy for eating disorders. New York: Guilford Press; 2008.
2. Fairburn CG, Cooper Z, Doll HA, et al. Enhanced cognitive behaviour therapy for adults with anorexia nervosa: a UK-Italy study. Behav Res Ther 2013;51:2–8.
3. National Institute for Health and Care Excellence. Eating Disorders: Recognition and Treatment (NG69). London: NICE; 2017.
4. Cooper Z, Fairburn CG. The evolution of "enhanced" cognitive behavior therapy for eating disorders: learning from treatment nonresponse. Cogn Behav Pract 2011;18:394–402.
5. Fairburn CG. The transdiagnostic view and cognitive behavioral therapy. In: Fairburn CG, editor. Cognitive behavior therapy and eating disorders. New York: Guilford Press; 2008. p. 7–22.
6. Byrne ME, Eichen DM, Fitzsimmons-Craft EE, et al. Perfectionism, emotion dysregulation, and affective disturbance in relation to clinical impairment in college-age women at high risk for or with eating disorders. Eat Behav 2016;23:131–6.
7. Agras WS, Rossiter EM, Arnow B, et al. Pharmacologic and cognitive-behavioral treatment for bulimia nervosa: a controlled comparison. Am J Psychiatry 1992; 149:82–7.
8. Agras WS, Walsh BT, Fairburn CG, et al. A multicenter comparison of cognitive-behavioral therapy and interpersonal psychotherapy for bulimia nervosa. Arch Gen Psychiatry 2000;57:459–66.
9. Fairburn CG, Bailey-Straebler S, Basden S, et al. A transdiagnostic comparison of enhanced cognitive behaviour therapy (CBT-E) and interpersonal psychotherapy in the treatment of eating disorders. Behav Res Ther 2015;70:64–71.
10. Fairburn CG, Jones R, Peveler RC, et al. Three psychological treatments for bulimia nervosa. Arch Gen Psychiatry 1991;48:463–9.
11. Mitchell JE, Agras WS, Crow S, et al. Stepped care and cognitive-behavioural therapy for bulimia nervosa: randomised trial. Br J Psychiatry 2011;198:391–7.
12. Wilfley DE, Agras WS, Telch CF, et al. Group cognitive-behavioral therapy and group interpersonal psychotherapy for the non-purging bulimic: a controlled comparison. J Consult Clin Psychol 1993;61:296–305.
13. Wilfley DE, Welch RR, Stein RI, et al. A randomized comparison of group cognitive-behavioral therapy and group interpersonal psychotherapy for the

treatment of overweight individuals with binge-eating disorder. Arch Gen Psychiatry 2002;59:713–21.

14. Wilson GT, Wilfley DE, Agras WS, et al. Psychological treatments of binge eating disorder. Arch Gen Psychiatry 2010;67:94–101.

15. Spielmans GI, Benish SG, Marin C, et al. Specificity of psychological treatments for bulimia nervosa and binge eating disorder? A meta-analysis of direct comparisons. Clin Psychol Rev 2013;33:460–9.

16. Grilo RM, Reas DL, Mitchell JE. Combining pharmacological and psychological treatments for binge eating disorder: current status, limitations, and future directions. Curr Psychiatry Rep 2016;18:55–60.

17. Shah N, Passi V, Bryson S, et al. Patterns of eating and abstinence in women treated for bulimia nervosa. Int J Eat Disord 2005;38:330–4.

18. Ellison JM, Simonich HK, Wonderlich SA, et al. Meal patterning in the treatment of bulimia nervosa. Eat Behav 2015;20:39–42.

19. Zendegui EA, West JA, Zandberg LJ. Binge eating frequency and regular eating adherence: the role of eating pattern in cognitive behavioral guided self-help. Eat Behav 2014;15:241–3.

20. Vall E, Wade T. Predictors of treatment outcome in individuals with eating disorders: a systematic review and meta-analysis. Int J Eat Disord 2015;48:946–71.

21. Agras WS, Crow SJ, Halmi KA, et al. Outcome predictors for the cognitive behavior treatment of bulimia nervosa: data from a multisite study. Am J Psychiatry 2000;157:1302–8.

22. Grilo CM, Masheb RM. Rapid response predicts binge eating and weight loss in binge eating disorder: findings from a controlled trial of orlistat with guided self-help cognitive behavioral therapy. Behav Res Ther 2007;45:2537–50.

23. Slade E, Keeney E, Mavranezouli I, et al. Treatments for bulimia nervosa: a network meta-analysis. Psychol Med 2018;48(16):2629–36.

24. Linardon J, Wade T, Garcia DP, et al. The efficacy of cognitive-behavioral therapy for eating disorders: a systematic meta-analysis. J Consult Clin Psychol 2017;85:1080–94.

25. Poulsen S, Lunn S, Daniel SF, et al. Psychotherapy or cognitive-behavioral therapy for bulimia nervosa. Am J Psychiatry 2014;171:109–16.

26. Stefinin A, Salzer S, Reich G, et al. Cognitive-behavioral and psychodynamic therapy in female adolescents with bulimia nervosa: a randomized controlled trial. J Am Acad Child Adolesc Psychiatry 2017;56:329–35.

27. Traviss-Turner GD, West RM, Hill AJ. Guided self-help for eating disorders: a systematic review and metaregression. Eur Eat Disord Rev 2017;25:148–64.

28. Wilson GT, Zandberg LJ. Cognitive-behavioral therapy guided self-help for eating disorders: effectiveness and scalability. Clin Psychol Rev 2012;32:343–57.

29. Fairburn CG. Overcoming binge eating. New York: Guilford Press; 1995.

30. Thompson-Brenner H, Shingleton RM, Thompson DR, et al. Focused vs. broad enhanced cognitive-behavioral therapy for bulimia nervosa with comorbid borderline personality: a randomized controlled trial. Int J Eat Disord 2016;49:36–49.

31. Schmidt U, Lee S, Beecham J, et al. A randomized controlled trial of family therapy and cognitive behavior therapy guided self-care for adolescents with bulimia nervosa and related disorders. Am J Psychiatry 2007;164:591–8.

32. Le Grange D, Lock J, Agras WS. Randomized clinical trial of family-based treatment and cognitive-behavioral therapy for adolescent bulimia nervosa. J Am Acad Child Adolesc Psychiatry 2015;54:886–94.

33. Blom TJ, Mingione CJ, Guerdjikova AI, et al. Placebo response in binge eating disorder: a pooled analysis of 10 clinical trials from one research group. Eur Eat Disord Rev 2014;22:140–6.
34. Palavras MA, Hay P, Filho CA, et al. The efficacy of psychological therapies in reducing weight and binge eating in people with bulimia nervosa and binge eating disorder who are overweight or obese-a critical synthesis and meta-analysis. Nutrients 2017;9:E299.
35. Agras WS, Telch CF, Arnow B, et al. Does interpersonal therapy help patients with binge eating disorder who fail to respond to cognitive-behavioral therapy? J Consult Clin Psychol 1995;63:356–60.
36. Galsworthy-Francis L, Allan S. Cognitive behavioural therapy for anorexia nervosa; a systematic review. Clin Psychol Rev 2014;34:54–72.
37. Hay P, Claudino A, Touyz S, et al. Individual psychological therapy in the outpatient treatment of adults with anorexia nervosa. Cochrane Database Syst Rev 2015;(7):CD003909.
38. Byrne S, Wade T, Hay P, et al. A randomized controlled trial of three psychological treatments for anorexia nervosa. Psychol Med 2017;29:2823–33.
39. Zeek A, Herpertz-Dahlmann B, Friederich HC, et al. Psychotherapeutic treatment for anorexia nervosa: a systematic review and network meta-analysis. Front Psychiatry 2018;1:158.
40. Grave RD, Calugi S, Doll HA, et al. Enhanced cognitive behaviour therapy for adolescents with anorexia nervosa: an alternative to family therapy? Behav Res Ther 2013;51:9–12.

Behavioral Interventions in the Treatment of Eating Disorders

Glenn Waller, DPhil[a],*, Bronwyn Raykos, PhD[b,1]

KEYWORDS

- Eating disorders • Behavior therapy • Anorexia nervosa • Bulimia nervosa
- Nutrition

KEY POINTS

- Nutritional change is key to the treatment of all eating disorders.
- Other behavioral methods also are important—in particular, exposure and skills development.
- Clinicians routinely fail to deliver on these key behavioral elements of therapy.

INTRODUCTION

Behavior therapy is rooted in the principles of learning (eg, operant and classical conditioning). Behavioral strategies are action based and highly focused, aiming to reduce or eliminate problematic behaviors through new learning. Behavioral interventions are present in a large proportion of evidence-based treatments of psychological disorders, although there is often a focus on the other elements of those treatments (eg, focusing on the cognitive rather than the behavioral methods). In relation to treatments of eating disorders, there has been limited consideration of the importance of behavioral interventions and learning principles. Are behavioral methods either necessary or sufficient to explain the outcome of evidence-based therapies for patients with eating disorders?

In its 2017 update, the National Institute for Health and Care Excellence[1] recommended a limited set of evidence-based psychological treatments of eating disorders, which included cognitive behavior therapy (CBT), family-based treatment

Disclosure Statement: The authors have no relationships or competing interests to declare.
[a] Department of Psychology, University of Sheffield, Cathedral Court, 1 Vicar Lane, Sheffield S1 2LT, UK; [b] Centre for Clinical Interventions, Perth, Western Australia, Australia
[1] Present address: 223 James Street, Northbridge, WA 6003, Australia.
* Corresponding author.
E-mail address: g.waller@sheffield.ac.uk

(FBT), and specialist supportive clinical management (SSCM)[a]. A common element of these treatments is a strong focus on using behavioral strategies to reduce eating disorder symptoms, with all interventions particularly focused on normalizing eating habits and weight. Each of these therapies integrates behavioral strategies with other elements, such as structural, systemic, and narrative interventions in FBT and cognitive strategies in CBT. Consequently, it is not clear which are the necessary components of each therapy. Understanding which components of each treatment are necessary is pertinent to the efficient and effective delivery of psychological therapies for any disorder. In other psychological disorders, it has been demonstrated that the behavioral elements of treatment are sufficient to generate most of the change that is attributed to the full therapy.[2-4] Few studies have dismantled treatment components to identify the most important mechanisms of change for patients with eating disorders. Therefore, the relative importance of behavioral interventions compared with other treatment components is currently poorly understood.

The value of behavioral strategies in reducing psychopathology in other disorders and the strong focus on behavioral strategies in effective therapies for eating disorders raises several important questions:

- Are behavioral strategies sufficient to drive the outcomes of evidence-based treatments of eating disorders?
- What are the key behavioral strategies that are necessary in treating eating disorders?
- By what mechanisms do behavioral strategies operate?

From the outset, it should be emphasized that definitive answers are not currently possible given the lack of true dismantling studies. It also should be stressed that behavioral interventions for eating disorders are not used simply to target eating disorder behaviors but also have the implicit and explicit targets of creating other changes (eg, modifying emotions and cognitions in CBT and modifying family interactions around the eating problems in FBT).

Given these questions and contextual factors in the literature, this article

1. Summarizes the literature on purely behavioral approaches for eating disorders
2. Identifies key behavioral interventions in evidence-based treatments of eating disorders
3. Considers the evidence regarding how those behavioral interventions work

Finally, the authors consider some of the clinician-level obstacles to implementation of behavioral methods

DO PURELY BEHAVIORAL APPROACHES WORK FOR EATING DISORDERS?

Behavioral strategies are commonly used in the treatment of eating disorders. For example, within inpatient units, operant conditioning techniques have been used to encourage patients with anorexia nervosa to eat and regain weight.[5] In eating disorder inpatient units in Germany, experts report routinely using behavioral contracts in the management of anorexia nervosa,[6,7] with the goal of motivating patients to gain weight by applying positive and negative consequences for the achievement or nonachievement of weight goals. The most frequently used positive consequences

---

[a] Although other treatments that include behavioral strategies have been researched (eg, dialectical behavior therapy, acceptance, and commitment therapy), their lower level of benefit[1] means that they are not be included in this article.

are the cessation of ward restriction (84%), hospital leave (83%), and the cessation of a liquid diet, whereas the most frequently used negative consequences were restriction to the ward (87%) and additional high-caloric nutrients (70%). Experts rated behavioral contracts as highly effective, although there currently is no empirical research examining that effectiveness, and the high rates of relapse after discharge from hospital suggest that behavioral interventions in isolation may not be sufficient to deliver recovery or sustained remission in isolation.

Cue exposure (exposing the individual to the characteristics of the feared object, such as the smell or taste of a binge food) also has been used to address the urge to binge in routine clinical practice. For example, in a small sample of nonresponders to pharmacologic treatment or CBT, cue exposure was associated with almost complete cessation of binge-eating and vomiting behaviors in individuals with bulimia nervosa that was sustained at long-term follow-up.[8] In routine practice, however, behavioral elements are usually integrated into a wider package of care, where their individual benefits cannot be assessed. Therefore, this article first focuses on pure behavior therapies for eating disorders. There is little evidence relating to such interventions for children and adolescents and almost nothing relating specifically to behavior therapies for binge-eating disorder or other atypical eating disorders in adulthood.

Behavioral Therapy for Bulimia Nervosa

When considering the outcome of behavioral therapy (BT) in isolation, the earliest studies to consider are those of Freeman and colleagues[9] and Fairburn and colleagues,[10,11] although others have been published more recently. The core elements in BT for bulimia nervosa are detailed in **Table 1**.

Fairburn compared BT to CBT and an interpersonal approach. Their behavioral approach is described as a "dismantled" form of CBT, focusing "exclusively on the normalization of eating habits."[10] In this therapy, the emphasis of the behavior change was on

Table 1
Elements of behavioral therapy, as used to treat bulimia nervosa and anorexia nervosa

| | Type of Therapy | Element of Intervention | | | Measurement Point | |
		Regularize Eating	Monitoring Eating	Systematic Desensitization	Effective by End of Therapy?	Effective at Follow-up?
Bulimia nervosa						
Freeman et al,[9] 1988	BT				++	Not known
Fairburn et al,[10,11] 1993 and 1995	BT				++	—
Barakat et al,[12] 2017	Dietary change (4 wk)				+	Not known
Anorexia nervosa						
Channon et al,[15] 1989	BT				++	++
McIntosh et al,[19] 2005	SSCM				++	++

- Regaining control over eating
- Establishing a regular pattern of eating
- Ceasing to diet

Although this purely behavioral approach, focused on normalization of eating habits, was associated with improvements by the end of therapy,[10] the results for BT were weaker than those for CBT and the interpersonal intervention. BT had higher rates of attrition during the therapy and lower effectiveness than CBT in the short and longer term. By the end of the 6-year follow-up, BT was performing far less well than the other therapies—probably no better than spontaneous recovery levels would have explained. This finding suggests that BT in isolation may not be sufficient to change eating disorder behaviors.

A similar approach has been presented,[12] based on dietary change (establishing a pattern of eating every 3 hours) and self-monitoring (recording food and drink intake and frequency of bulimic behaviors). Their intervention was conducted over only 4 weeks, meaning that the effects were relatively small. The level of effect, however, was substantially smaller than that achieved by the first 4 weeks of CBT,[13] suggesting that BT in isolation may be less effective in reducing symptoms of bulimia nervosa than therapies that combine behavioral and cognitive strategies. Another related behavioral approach to treating bulimia nervosa (nutrition, feedback on pacing of eating, and thermoregulation) is stated to have positive results.[14] Although a large number of patients have been treated using this approach, the substantial methodological problems in the studies (eg, lack of control groups, nonreplicability, handling of missing data, and omission of very large numbers of patients from the sample included in the analyses) mean, however, that the evidence of outcomes is relatively weak. Thus, it seems that a nutrition-based behavioral intervention in isolation is of limited utility in treating bulimia nervosa.

In contrast, Freeman and colleagues[9] described a form of BT for bulimia nervosa that was slightly broader than that Fairburn and colleagues,[11,12] because it incorporated graded tasks and relaxation training (ie, systematic desensitization) as well as regularization of eating and self-monitoring. Unlike Fairburn and colleagues' outcomes (discussed previously), BT had similar outcomes to those of CBT and tended to have a lower attrition rate across the course of therapy. The loss to follow-up in this study means that it cannot be concluded that the outcomes were sustained equally for all therapies. This study highlights the possibility, however, that behavioral interventions that more thoroughly address long-standing fear-based learning might perform at least as well as CBT at post-treatment.

To summarize, in treating bulimia nervosa, behavioral strategies based primarily on nutritional changes are effective in the short term but are not sufficient to generate the level of remission and recovery that are found in CBT.[9] Although it is likely that behavioral interventions focused on nutritional change and normalizing eating habits are necessary, it is possible that exposure-based elements or cognitive elements are also needed to enhance such nutritional elements.

Behavioral Therapy for Anorexia Nervosa

Table 1 shows the key studies of BT for anorexia nervosa and the behavioral techniques involved.[b] The first controlled study that examined the impact of purely

---

[b] Because of the substantial methodological issues with Bergh and colleagues, article,[14] as discussed previously, that study is not included in this review and does not contribute to the conclusions.

behavioral approaches on anorexia nervosa compared the outcome of BT and CBT.[15] Their behavioral approach included nutritional changes, using a graded approach to feared foods combined with relaxation components (ie, systematic desensitization, rather than the more effective approach of graded exposure). The outcomes for BT and CBT both tended to be positive relative to treatment as usual and were equivalent across the 2 therapies, even though attendance at BT was poorer. The conclusion reached was that adding cognitive elements to BT did not have measurable benefits for anorexia nervosa. The small sample size in each condition (n = 8), however, leaves the possibility that the lack of significant differences is attributable to low power. Further replication studies are needed to assess whether these results are generalizable. The investigators also noted that the lack of significant differences between the CBTs and behavioral treatments may be because directly manipulating cognitive processes using techniques, such as cognitive restructuring, is unnecessary because behavioral change is mediated by cognitive factors—that is, both treatments might work via the same mechanisms of change.

A second behavioral approach that has been used successfully with adults with anorexia nervosa is SSCM.[16] SSCM's only behavioral, action-based technique is focusing the patient on the need for weight gain and normalization of eating. Thus, the key behavioral method used is nutritional change, as with Fairburn and colleagues'[10,11] BT approach to bulimia nervosa. The value of the behavioral strategies within SSCM for anorexia nervosa is demonstrated by its outcomes with this clinical group. In several trials to date,[17–21] SSCM has proved at least as effective as other therapies (including CBT, Maudsley Model of Anorexia Nervosa Treatment for Adults [MANTRA], and interpersonal psychotherapy) in the treatment of anorexia nervosa (including atypical cases), in the short term and longer term. Thus, it seems that SSCM is a behavioral approach that is at least as effective for anorexia nervosa as other interventions, such as CBT. The support with life issues element of SSCM, however, is less clearly defined,[16] so it is possible that there are elements here that are not entirely behavioral.

To summarize, although outcomes across treatments are weaker for anorexia nervosa than they are for bulimia nervosa, behavioral approaches to anorexia nervosa seem as effective as broader approaches. The question that arises in consequence is whether more complex forms of therapy should be implemented when BT may be at least as effective as (and easier to deliver than) those other approaches.

Behavioral Therapy for Eating and Feeding Disorders of Childhood and Adolescence

The most strongly recommended treatments of children and adolescents with eating disorders are family based, although CBT can be used in some cases.[1] Although these approaches all include substantial focus on nutrition and behavioral change, they are embedded within wider systemic and cognitive approaches, making the behavioral element impossible to isolate. The literature on the use of BT with these cases is also made harder to interpret as a result of inconsistent definitions used across the field.[22] Changes in categorization have been operationalized under the *Diagnostic and Statistical Manual of Mental Disorders* (Fifth Edition) (*DSM-5*).[23] The recency of that definitional change means that research into the treatment of the new categories is in its infancy. Although there are some promising treatments in development for such cases,[24] few are purely behavioral in nature.

Considering the evidence for such disorders under the less well-defined categories that preceded *DSM-5*, some behavioral strategies (eg, nutritional change, stimulus control, extinction, and contingency management) are effective in the treatment of young children with feeding disorders.[25] Similarly, it has been suggested that exposure-based methods should be used for selective eating across the age span.[26] The conclusions that can be reached about the role of BT in younger cases, however, are limited.

Summary

At present, the evidence for BT as an approach to eating disorders is limited but suggests different responses according to the nature of the disorders. Behavioral methods (particularly focused on nutrition) might seem as effective as other therapies for anorexia nervosa. Given that the literature has several limitations (eg, lack of extended follow-up and high relapse rates post-hospitalization), however, it might be premature to suggest that BT is sufficient as a treatment of anorexia nervosa. The evidence is more mixed when considering treatment of bulimia nervosa, where it seems that simple nutritional change is necessary but not sufficient to effect positive, sustained outcomes and that exposure techniques might be necessary to maximize the effects of nutritional change. It also seems that BTs are effective with some childhood eating disorders, but further research is needed to support that case, especially given recent diagnostic changes. This is only a small part of the evidence regarding treatment of eating disorders, however, and many of the existing treatment packages for eating disorders contain substantial behavioral strategies. The key behavioral strategies that are commonly used in that way are discussed later.

KEY BEHAVIORAL STRATEGIES IN THE TREATMENT OF EATING DISORDERS

When considering behavioral elements in the evidence-based treatment of eating disorders, it should be remembered that those elements are most commonly found as components of full-therapy protocols, such as CBT,[27,28] FBT,[29,30] SSCM,[16] and

Table 2
Core behavioral techniques used in evidence-based therapies

Behavioral Technique	Examples of General Roles	Found in
Change in eating patterns	• Enhances flexible thinking • Mood stabilization • Weight regain and stabilization	• FBT • CBT-ED • MANTRA • SSCM • BT
Exposure with response prevention	• Reduce anxiety • Reduce avoidant behaviors (eg, restriction and not using mirrors) • Reduce safety behaviors (eg, bingeing to block emotional states and vomiting to avoid feared weight gain)	• CBT-ED • MANTRA • BT (some)
Behavioral experiments	• Testing and changing cognitions • Reduces beliefs about the uncontrollability of weight gain • Reduces belief in value of body checking and comparison • Enhancement of self-esteem • Reduction in beliefs about the value of perfectionist style	• CBT-ED
Behavioral skills training	• Meal planning • Parental management skills	• FBT • CBT-ED • BT • SSCM

MANTRA.[31] The techniques are not always labeled as such within the specific therapy protocol, although they serve the functions outlined. The most important of those techniques are outlined in **Table 2**, along with examples of their use and whether they are found in different therapies. These techniques are used differently across therapies, as discussed later.

Normalizing Eating Patterns and Weight

A majority of evidence-based therapies for eating disorders stress nutritional change as necessary, but they differ in the timing of change. For example, in underweight cases, Fairburn[27] stresses nutritional behavior change as an early focus in CBT-enhanced for non-underweight and underweight patients but only emphasizes the need for weight gain later. In contrast, Waller and colleagues[13,28] emphasize the need for nutritional behavior change and weight regain from the outset, regardless of diagnosis. Similarly, nutritional change is described as a target from the outset in MANTRA for anorexia nervosa.[31] In all these approaches, however, changing eating structure and content to ensure weight gain and weight maintenance are stressed as key skills.

Skills Training

The development and implementation of practical skills can assist patients who have a long history of an eating disorder and a consequent loss of self-esteem and confidence. The development of such skills is a central part of all the evidence-based therapies discussed in this article (eg, the parental skills needed to manage behavioral change in FBT and the practical skills of planning, shopping, and food preparation that are stressed in SSCM). The support of a wide range of professionals (eg, dietitians and occupational therapists) can be valuable.

Exposure and Avoidance of Safety Behaviors

Exposure is a core element of CBT for eating disorders (CBT-ED) and BT, although it is not always explicitly detailed in the relevant protocols. The changes to eating that are stressed in other effective therapies, however, mean that exposure takes place there, too. In CBT-ED and BT, such exposure is used to reduce anxiety and fear. Through sustained exposure to the feared object (eg, food or seeing one's body), the individual learns that the feared negative outcome (eg, weight gain) does not occur. As well as changes in eating patterns, exposure is used to address other important maintaining factors, such as body avoidance, binge eating, purging, and avoidance of being weighed.

Although most exposure is delivered using a habituation paradigm (using hierarchy-based methods), developments in the anxiety literature suggest that this approach is not as effective as an approach based on inhibitory learning.[32] Consequently, it has been suggested that inhibitory learning should be used to underpin the use of exposure in working with eating disorders.[33] Such a goal means that clinicians should aim to ensure that a patient's anxiety is maximized (rather than increased slowly between sessions, using a hierarchy) and that the exposure should be practiced in as wide a range of settings as possible, to maximize and deepen the patient's learning. To date, this approach has only been reported in 1 form of CBT-ED,[13,34] but that 10-session version (CBT-T) has demonstrated promisingly rapid results that are sustained to follow-up. The form of exposure to be used in future versions of CBT-ED and other therapies merits consideration.

Behavioral Experiments

The behavioral experiments technique addresses cognitive distortions and errors and is exclusive to CBT-ED. Behavioral experiments are more commonly used later in therapy, because it can be important to reduce anxiety levels before an individual can reliably make a single change to learn its consequences. Experiments can be set up earlier in CBT-ED, however, to help patients learn that their weight does not increase uncontrollably, as they believe will be the case.[35] Behavioral experiments are used in different ways in the different forms of CBT-ED, for example:

- Fairburn[27] stresses the use of such experiments to modify beliefs related to self-esteem and perfectionism
- Waller and colleagues[28] also use such experiments to
  - Correct specific beliefs about the impact on weight of changes in energy balance (eg, introducing specific foods and changing exercise levels)
  - Reduce body-related behaviors (in particular checking and comparison)
- Waller and colleagues[36] have recently suggested that clinicians should aim to maximize the level and speed of learning for patients by raising their anxiety prior to making predictions (eg, discussing eating patterns in depth immediately before predicting weight gain), so that patients' predictions can be shown to be more incorrect.

Mechanisms Underlying the Effects of Behavioral Interventions for Eating Disorders

The evidence, discussed previously, makes a clear case that behavioral techniques are necessary for the effective treatment of eating disorders and their different symptoms. The mechanisms of change, however, are not always clear. Behavioral experiments are usually assumed to operate by changing cognitions,[37] but it is also possible that there is a mood-change element. Similarly, exposure is assumed to be a method for reducing affect, but there is likely to be cognitive change too. Despite its long history, how exposure works is still not clear, with long-standing suggestions, including habituation and extinction, and more recent explanations centering on inhibitory learning processes.[33] What is more clear is that the behavioral changes relating to nutritional balance have their widespread impact via enhancing mood stability and positive affect, cognitive flexibility, biological safety, and interpersonal/social functioning.[38,39] These changes, however, are likely to be complex and interactive rather than distinct, explaining the extent of the effects of nutritional balance.

Even though the learning and biological mechanisms of behavioral change are not always clearly understood, a key feature of behavioral strategies is their transparency. These methods are highly observable, discrete, and focused, so the therapist and the patient can observe their impact clearly. That transparency of effect means that learning can be maximized, with clear causality established. When patients learn the effect of behavioral change, they can learn to change their everyday behaviors in an adaptive way; when therapists learn the effect of behavioral change, they can carry it over to future patients with greater confidence.

A CAVEAT: THE ROLE OF THE CLINICIAN IN THE DELIVERY OF BEHAVIORAL METHODS

Although the evidence, discussed previously, clearly shows that behavioral methods have a necessary role in the treatment of eating disorders, no therapy has the potential to help patients if it is not used. With that in mind, it is important to remember that clinicians rarely use treatment protocols in the field of eating disorders[40,41] and report relatively low use of key behavioral methods. For example, clinicians who report that they use CBT-ED describe using structured eating regularly with approximately only half of their patients and using behavioral experiments and exposure with approximately only a third.[42,43] This failure to use behavioral methods is not confined to CBT-ED, as shown by the reported reluctance of clinicians to use nutritional change and other key methods in SSCM, MANTRA, and FBT.[16,31,44] Possibly more worrying is that clinicians' own anxiety levels are predictive of whether they will use structured eating, exposure, and weighing.[42,43,45] This impact of clinician anxiety is known outside of the field of eating disorders and has resulted in the suggestion that clinicians' own anxiety levels should be addressed in supervision, using role play.

SUMMARY

In treating eating disorders, it is clear that

- The field does not have the necessary dismantling studies to demonstrate which elements are critical in explaining the outcomes of effective therapies.
- Behavioral components are definitely necessary, across therapies and diagnoses, to get the strongest outcomes.
- In anorexia nervosa, the central behavioral strategy of nutritional change seems the most important aspect of evidence-based treatments.
- A range of behavioral techniques is valuable in the treatment of eating disorders. Although behavioral methods are inherent in some techniques used in other evidence-based therapies, they are more overtly planned into CBT-ED and BT.
- Even within CBT-ED, the methods are used differently, reflecting disparate models.
- Despite their being key to CBT-ED and other therapies, clinicians do not always use behavioral methods and are less likely to do so in response to their own anxiety levels.

REFERENCES

1. National Institute for Health and Care Excellence. Eating disorders: recognition and treatment. London: National Institute for Health and Care Excellence; 2017.
2. Jacobson NS, Dobson KS, Truax PA, et al. A component analysis of cognitive-behavioral treatment for depression. J Consult Clin Psychol 1996;64:295–304.
3. Ougrin D. Efficacy of exposure versus cognitive therapy in anxiety disorders: Systematic review and meta-analysis. BMC Psychiatry 2011;11:200.
4. Parker ZJ, Waller G, Gonzalez-Salas Duhne P, et al. The role of exposure in treatment of anxiety disorders: a meta-analysis. Int J Psychol Psychol Ther 2018;18: 111–41.
5. Leitenberg H, Agras WS, Thomson LE. A sequential analysis of the effect of selective positive reinforcement in modifying anorexia nervosa. Behav Res Ther 1968;6:211–8.
6. Ziser K, Giel KE, Resmark G, et al. Contingency contracts for weight gain of patients with anorexia nervosa in inpatient therapy: practice styles of specialized centers. J Clin Med 2018;7:215.
7. Ziser K, Resmark G, Giel KE, et al. The effectiveness of contingency management in the treatment of patients with anorexia nervosa: a systematic review. Eur Eat Disord Rev 2018;26:379–93.

8. Toro J, Cervera M, Garriga N, et al. Cue exposure in the treatment of resistant bulimia nervosa. Int J Eat Disord 2003;34:227–34.
9. Freeman CPL, Barry F, Dunkeld-Turnbull J, et al. Controlled trial of psychotherapy for bulimia nervosa. BMJ 1988;296:521–5.
10. Fairburn CG, Jones R, Peveler RC, et al. Psychotherapy and bulimia nervosa. Longer-term effects of interpersonal psychotherapy, behavior therapy, and cognitive behavior therapy. Arch Gen Psychiatry 1993;50:419–28.
11. Fairburn CG, Norman PA, Welch SL, et al. A prospective study of outcome in bulimia nervosa and the long-term effects of three psychological treatments. Arch Gen Psychiatry 1995;52:304–12.
12. Barakat S, Maguire S, Surgenor L, et al. The role of regular eating and self-monitoring in the treatment of bulimia nervosa: a pilot study of an online guided self-help CBT program. Behav Sci 2017;26:7.
13. Waller G, Tatham M, Turner H, et al. A 10-session cognitive-behavioral therapy (CBT-T) for eating disorders: outcomes from a case series of non-underweight adult patients. Int J Eat Disord 2018;51:262–9.
14. Bergh C, Callmar M, Danemar S, et al. Effective treatment of eating disorders: Results at multiple sites. Behav Neurosci 2013;127:878–89.
15. Channon S, De Silva P, Hemsley D, et al. Controlled trial of cognitive-behavioural and behavioural treatment of anorexia nervosa. Behav Res Ther 1989;27:529–35.
16. Jordan J, McIntosh VVW, Bulik CM. Specialist supportive clinical management for anorexia nervosa. In: Wade T, editor. Encyclopaedia of eating and feeding disorders. New York: Springer; 2017.
17. Byrne S, Wade T, Hay P, et al. A randomised controlled trial of three psychological treatments for anorexia nervosa. Psychol Med 2017;47:2823–33.
18. Carter FA, Jordan J, McIntosh VV, et al. The long-term efficacy of three psychotherapies for anorexia nervosa. A randomized controlled trial. Int J Eat Disord 2011;44:647–54.
19. McIntosh VV, Jordan J, Carter FA, et al. Three psychotherapies for anorexia nervosa: a randomized controlled trial. Am J Psychiatry 2005;162:741–7.
20. Schmidt U, Magill N, Renwick B, et al. The Maudsley Outpatient Study of Treatments for Anorexia Nervosa and Related Conditions (MOSAIC): comparison of the Maudsley Model of Anorexia Nervosa Treatment for Adults (MANTRA) with Specialist Supportive Clinical Management (SSCM) in outpatients with broadly defined anorexia nervosa: a randomized controlled trial. J Consult Clin Psychol 2015;83:796–807.
21. Touyz S, le Grange D, Lacey H, et al. Treating severe and enduring anorexia nervosa: a randomized controlled trial. Psychol Med 2013;43:2501–11.
22. Bryant-Waugh R, Markham L, Kreipe RE, et al. Feeding and eating disorders in childhood. Int J Eat Disord 2010;43:98–111.
23. American Psychiatric Association. Diagnostic and statistical manual of mental disorders: DSM-V. 5th edition. Washington, DC: American Psychiatric Association; 1994.
24. Thomas JJ, Wons OB, Eddy KT. Cognitive-behavioral treatment of avoidant/restrictive food intake disorder. Curr Opin Psychiatry 2018;31:425–30.
25. Lukens CT, Silverman AH. Systematic review of psychological interventions for pediatric feeding problems. J Pediatr Psychol 2014;39:903–17.
26. Nicholls D, Christie D, Randall L, et al. Selective eating: symptom, disorder or normal variant. Clin Child Psychol Psychiatry 2001;6:257–70.
27. Fairburn CG. Cognitive behavior therapy and eating disorders. New York: Guilford; 2008.

28. Waller G, Cordery H, Corstorphine E, et al. Cognitive-behavioral therapy for the eating disorders: a comprehensive treatment guide. Cambridge (United Kingdom): Cambridge University Press; 2007.
29. Lock J, LeGrange D. Treatment manual for anorexia nervosa: a family-based approach. 2nd edition. New York: Guilford; 2013.
30. LeGrange D, Lock J. Treating bulimia in adolescents: a family-based approach. New York: Guilford; 2007.
31. Schmidt U, Wade TD, Treasure J. The maudsley model of anorexia nervosa treatment for adults (MANTRA): development, key features, and preliminary evidence. J Cogn Psychother 2014;28:48–71.
32. Craske MG, Treanor M, Conway CC, et al. Maximizing exposure therapy: an inhibitory learning approach. Behav Res Ther 2014;58:10–23.
33. Reilly ER, Anderson LM, Gorrell S, et al. Expanding exposure-based interventions for eating disorders. Int J Eat Disord 2017;50:1137–41.
34. Pellizzer M, Waller G, Wade TD. Ten-session cognitive behaviour therapy for eating disorders: Outcomes from a pragmatic pilot study of Australian non-underweight patients. Clinical Psychologist, in press.
35. Waller G, Mountford VA. Weighing patients within cognitive-behavioural therapy for eating disorders: How, when and why. Behav Res Ther 2015;70:1–10.
36. Waller G, Turner H, Tatham M, et al. Brief cognitive behavioural therapy for non-underweight patients: CBT-T for eating disorders. Hove (United Kingdom): Routledge, in press.
37. Beck AT, Rush AJ, Shaw BF, et al. Cognitive therapy of depression. New York: Guilford; 1979.
38. Waller G, Evans J, Pugh M. Food for thought: a pilot study of the pros and cons of changing eating patterns within cognitive-behavioural therapy for the eating disorders. Behav Res Ther 2013;51:519–25.
39. Keys A, Brozek J, Henschel A, et al. The biology of human starvation. Minneapolis (MN): University of Minnesota Press; 1950.
40. Tobin DL, Banker JD, Weisberg L, et al. I know what you did last summer (and it was not CBT): A factor analytic model of international psychotherapeutic practice in the eating disorders. Int J Eat Disord 2007;40:754–7.
41. Waller G. Treatment protocols for eating disorders: clinicians' attitudes, concerns, adherence and difficulties delivering evidence-based psychological interventions. Curr Psychiatry Rep 2016;18(4):36.
42. Mulkens S, de Vos C, de Graaff A, et al. To deliver or not to deliver cognitive behavioral therapy for eating disorders: replication and extension of our understanding of why therapists fail to do what they should do. Behav Res Ther 2018;106:57–63.
43. Waller G, Stringer H, Meyer C. What cognitive-behavioral techniques do therapists report using when delivering cognitive-behavioral therapy for the eating disorders? J Consult Clin Psychol 2012;80:171–5.
44. Kosmerly S, Waller G, Robinson AL. Clinician adherence to guidelines in the delivery of family-based therapy for eating disorders. Int J Eat Disord 2015;48: 223–9.
45. Levita L, Salas Duhne PG, Girling C, et al. Facets of clinicians' anxiety and the delivery of cognitive-behaviour therapy. Behav Res Ther 2016;77:157–61.

Family-based Treatment of Eating Disorders
A Narrative Review

Sasha Gorrell, PhD[a], Katherine Loeb, PhD[b],
Daniel Le Grange, PhD[c,d,*]

KEYWORDS

- Family-based treatment • Family intervention • Eating disorders • Anorexia nervosa
- Bulimia nervosa

KEY POINTS

- Current best practices for eating disorder treatment in adolescence and young adulthood include family-based interventions.
- Although evidence is gathering, there remains a paucity of randomized clinical trials for eating disorders aside from anorexia nervosa.
- Future efforts in family-based eating disorder treatment must include a focus on dissemination and implementation.

Eating disorders (EDs) are pernicious illnesses that are associated with significant psychiatric and medical morbidity and mortality,[1] considerable distress and impairment,[2] marked caregiver burden,[3] and high treatment costs.[4] Because EDs commonly onset in adolescence and young adulthood,[2] and with consistent evidence that early intervention results in the most promising treatment outcomes,[5] an increasing amount of research has been devoted to the treatment of adolescent EDs. Although still less researched than adult presentation of EDs, the historical record of adolescent ED treatment over the last half-century principally supports family therapy.[6,7] Current published clinical guidelines recommend an ED-specific family therapy as the first-line treatment

Disclosure: Dr S. Gorrell is supported by the National Institutes of Health T32 MH018261; Dr K. Loeb receives royalties from Routledge and is a faculty member of and consultant for the Training Institute for Child and Adolescent Eating Disorders; Dr D. Le Grange receives royalties from Guilford Press and Routledge and is codirector of the Training Institute for Child and Adolescent Eating Disorders, LLC.

[a] Department of Psychiatry, University of California, San Francisco, 401 Parnassus Avenue, San Francisco, CA 94143, USA; [b] School of Psychology, Fairleigh Dickinson University, 1000 River Road (T-WH1-01), Teaneck, NJ 07666, USA; [c] Eating Disorders Program, Department of Psychiatry, University of California, San Francisco, 401 Parnassus Avenue, San Francisco, CA 94143, USA; [d] The University of Chicago, Chicago, IL, USA
* Corresponding author. 401 Parnassus Avenue, San Francisco, CA 94143.
E-mail address: Daniel.LeGrange@ucsf.edu

Psychiatr Clin N Am 42 (2019) 193–204
https://doi.org/10.1016/j.psc.2019.01.004

of adolescents with anorexia nervosa (AN) and as a recommended treatment of adolescents with bulimia nervosa (BN).[8] The number of treatment trials for adolescent AN has slowly grown over the last few decades[9] and, more recently, family interventions include protocols extending to new populations and diagnoses, including BN.[10–12] This narrative review summarizes existing family-based approaches to the treatment of adolescent EDs, integrating recent research findings. This article also includes discussion of methods, both current and proposed, that expand and adapt current family-based approaches in efforts to improve the breadth and scope of ED treatment in adolescence and young adulthood.

FAMILY ROLE AND ENGAGEMENT IN EATING DISORDER TREATMENT

Historically, AN treatment excluded parental involvement in both diagnosis and intervention because parents were erroneously conceptualized as a causal factor in the pathogenesis of the ED.[13,14] A philosophic and evidence-based shift away from an emphasis on family responsibility in the cause of ED has allowed parents to be actively involved in the course of treatment[13,15] and to be viewed as a vital resource in aiding the young persons in the process of recovery.[16] Further, a broader understanding of family dynamics that develop in the context of an ED includes not only the ways in which the disorder negatively affects the patient and family but also how the ED may be partially maintained within the family's structural system.[17] At present, families are usually incorporated into the treatment of adolescents with AN,[9] and such involvement has been shown to significantly reduce psychological and medical morbidity, as well as decrease treatment attrition rates.[14] As such, and despite the paucity of family-based intervention trials for adolescent BN,[10] it is likely that treatment of transdiagnostic EDs in adolescence, beyond AN, may benefit from consistent family involvement.

The first randomized clinical trial (RCT) for AN that involved parents showed that family therapy was superior to individual psychotherapy at posthospitalization for adolescents with fewer than 3 years' duration of illness.[18] In the years since, family therapy for adolescent AN (treatment manual available at www.national. slam.nhs.uk/wp-content/uploads/2011/11/Maudsley-Service-Manual-for-Child-and-Adolescent-Eating-Disorders-July-2016.pdf) and family-based treatment (FBT), with treatment manuals corresponding to adolescent AN[19] and BN,[20] have emerged as the most promising treatments for medically stable adolescent ED presentations. This article, as a reflection of the larger body of research available on tested treatment protocols, focuses primarily on FBT.

FBT is characterized by an agnostic stance toward the cause and pathogenesis of the ED, along with the overarching tenet that parents are the most influential resource in their offspring's recovery. In initial stages of treatment, FBT mobilizes parental resources in weight restoration, as well as in disrupting the cycle of ED behaviors. FBT therapists serve as expert consultants to the families, supporting parents to assume ultimate responsibility for guiding their child through recovery. FBT engages parents by directing their parental capacities and instincts toward the ED target, positively shaping parents' effectiveness, and releasing them from worry that their efforts will erode family relationships or exacerbate the illness. As weight restoration and behavioral symptom resolution are facilitated, less parental authority is typically required and parents may gradually restore autonomy over eating to the adolescent. As the child returns to age-appropriate functioning, therapeutic focus can shift to typical adolescent developmental issues that were interrupted by the onset and course of the ED.

FAMILY-BASED TREATMENT OF ANOREXIA NERVOSA

FBT has been systematically studied in 8 RCTs, 6 of which have focused on AN, and this has provided a strong evidence base supporting the use of manualized FBT for adolescents with this illness. In the first RCT to use the FBT-AN manual, 121 adolescents with AN were randomized to either FBT or individual adolescent-focused therapy (AFT).[21] The primary outcome variable in this study was full remission, defined as reaching greater than or equal to 95% of expected body weight (%EBW), and achieving an eating disorder examination (EDE)[22] global score within 1 standard deviation (SD) of community norms. The investigators found no differences between the two groups at end of treatment, but significantly more patients receiving FBT had achieved full remission at 6-month (FBT 40% vs AFT 18%) and 12-month (FBT 49% vs AFT 23%) follow-up.

To delineate more precisely how the family, and parents specifically, may function within FBT, a multisite trial with 164 adolescents was conducted comparing FBT with systemic family therapy (SFT).[23] In SFT, difficulties such as AN are not thought to arise in individuals themselves but, instead, to develop within the relationships, interactions, and language in a given family system. Thus with this approach, the focus of treatment is on the family system, and normalization of eating and weight is not a specific focus of treatment unless raised by the family. Findings did not indicate significant differences between treatment groups in weight at end of treatment or 1-year follow-up. However, those receiving FBT gained weight significantly faster than those receiving SFT, and significantly fewer participants in FBT were hospitalized.

To evaluate differential effects of shorter-term versus longer-term FBT, in a study of 86 adolescents diagnosed with AN, participants were randomly assigned to either a 6-month (10 sessions) or a 12-month (20 sessions) duration of treatment and evaluated at the end of 1 year using the EDE.[24] Main outcomes in this study were between-group comparisons of EDE scores, and change in body mass index (BMI). Results indicated that a short-term course of FBT seems to be as effective as a long-term course for adolescents with AN. However, post hoc analyses suggest that individuals with more severe eating-related obsessive cognitions, or from nonintact or single-parent families, might benefit from longer treatment.

A trial investigating the impact of early weight gain on treatment outcomes enrolled 82 adolescents with AN who received either brief hospitalization for medical stabilization versus longer hospitalization for weight restoration to 90% EBW.[25] Following discharge, both groups received 20 sessions of FBT. Results indicated that weight gain greater than 1.8 kg at session 4 of FBT predicted greater %EBW as well as remission status at end of FBT and at 12-month follow-up. Notably, this early weight gain indicator predicted remission, whereas treatment arm randomization did not add significantly to the model. These findings underscore the importance of early weight gain, and also indicate that longer hospitalization is not required to enhance the effectiveness of FBT treatment of AN.

Taken together, these trials support the use of FBT for AN, over and above other forms of therapy, but also suggest that study of FBT-AN should include adaptations to specifically address predictors (eg, early weight gain) that may affect treatment outcomes. Other trials comparing standard conjoint FBT with a separate version of this treatment, called parent-focused therapy (PFT),[26] as well as with an adaptive/augmented format of FBT,[27] are discussed in depth later in this article in relation to specific treatment moderators.

FAMILY-BASED TREATMENT OF BULIMIA NERVOSA

Although prevalence estimates for adolescent BN are consistently higher than adolescent AN,[2] there is a limited amount of research evaluating treatment outcomes in this population.[28] To date, there have been 3 randomized controlled trials specifically evaluating treatment efficacy of FBT for BN. In a trial comparing an adaptation of family therapy for AN for use with individuals with BN, 85 adolescents with BN or eating disorder not otherwise specified were randomized to FT or to self-guided cognitive behavior therapy (CBT).[29] Considered a first line of treatment of adults with BN,[30] CBT in this trial was self-guided and supported by a health care professional. Primary outcomes were abstinence from binge eating and vomiting following 6 months of treatment, and at 12-month follow-up; secondary outcomes included attitudinal bulimic symptoms, and treatment cost. Results indicated that patients receiving self-guided CBT had significant reductions in binge eating at 6 months but these differences disappeared at follow-up. Further, there were no differences between groups in purging behavior or attitudinal symptoms. Direct cost of care was reduced in CBT, but groups did not differ across other cost categories. Findings suggest that self-guided CBT might be superior in achieving abstinence from binge eating more quickly compared with a family therapy approach, but these effects are not lasting.

With a manualized approach to family treatment of BN, a trial comparing FBT-BN with supportive psychotherapy (SPT) in 80 participants (aged 12–19 years) with a Diagnostic and Statistical Manual of Mental Disorders, Fourth Edition (DSM-IV) diagnosis of BN or partial BN (ie, those who endorsed binge and purge episodes averaging once per week over 6 months) were randomized to 1 of these 2 treatments, each for 20 sessions over 6 months.[31] SPT is a nondirective treatment that does not involve specific active therapeutic elements, and as a general treatment was considered comparable with what would be received in the community. Based on FBT-AN, FBT-BN also takes an agnostic stance about the cause of the ED, externalizes the illness, and empowers parents to disrupt maladaptive eating and compensatory behavior. However, compared with this treatment's AN format, FBT-BN takes the stance that this disorder is perhaps experienced as more ego-dystonic than is AN, and that most adolescents with BN are developmentally more on track than their AN counterparts. Therefore, FBT-BN allows for greater adolescent participation in the treatment process than is typically the case for AN. Results of this trial indicated that FBT-BN had significantly higher rates of abstinence from binge eating and purging episodes (39% vs 18%) at end of treatment; across both groups, the rate of abstinence declined when assessed at 12-month follow-up (29% and 10%, respectively).

In another trial, CBT was adapted for adolescents with BN (CBT-A) and compared with FBT-BN.[32] In this study, 109 adolescents (aged 12–18 years) with a DSM-IV diagnosis of BN or partial BN (as defined previously) were randomized to 1 of these 2 treatments, each for 18 sessions over 6 months. CBT-A is primarily an individual therapy that focuses on reducing dieting and changing distorted behaviors and cognitions related to shape and weight. Adaptations to CBT that were unique to CBT-A included exploration of developmental challenges, and parent collateral sessions that included psychoeducation for caregivers about BN. FBT-BN was delivered with the approach described earlier. Findings indicated that abstinence from binge eating and purging episodes at the end of treatment was significantly higher for FBT-BN than CBT-A (39.4% vs 19.7%). At 6-month follow-up, abstinence rates for both groups continued to improve but remained significantly different in favor of FBT (44% and 25.4% respectively); abstinence rates between the two groups did not differ statistically at 12-month follow-up (49% vs 32%).

Taken together, these trials provide provisional, but strikingly robust, support for the use of FBTs in the treatment of adolescent BN. In particular, the 2 trials described here comparing the efficacy of a manualized FBT-BN with another distinct and active treatment (SPT and CBT-A, respectively) increase the efficiency within the study design in determining the superiority of this intervention relative to other established standard-of-care treatments.[33] This outcome is notable in contrast with the increased number of RCTs that have evaluated the efficacy of FBT in adolescents with AN, with only 1 having compared FBT-AN with an active treatment.[27] Therefore, it might be concluded that, although much research remains to be conducted in adolescent treatment of BN, the robust nature of current evidence rivals, and may even supersede, the efficacy established for FBT-AN.

EXPANSION OF FAMILY-BASED TREATMENT

In the years following that initial trial, FBT-AN has been considerably expanded to address new populations, developmental stages, and diagnoses. In addition, it has been modified to improve its dissemination ease and reach. Although much of this work is nascent, what is described here shows notable expansion efforts, including in telehealth, which may greatly improve accessibility to specialty treatment. Other ways in which FBT may be improved are in changes to format specific to engaging with multiple families simultaneously, and in application transdiagnostically across EDs and beyond the traditional adolescent age group.

Telehealth Format

The concentration of FBT-trained therapists in primarily urban centers suggests that the use of telehealth in the delivery of FBT has the capacity to vastly increase access to this therapy for many patient populations. Recent work has investigated the feasibility and preliminary effect size of FBT for adolescents with AN delivered via a telehealth platform.[34,35] Treatment outcome was determined using percentage median BMI (mBMI), and the EDE. Findings indicate that mBMI significantly improved from baseline to end of treatment, and that this improvement was retained at 6-month follow-up. Similar results were achieved for the EDE global score, providing preliminary evidence that FBT via telehealth yields satisfactory clinical outcomes and warrants further investigation. Future confirmation of the success of this particular format in a larger treatment trial may ultimately allow more families to secure access to greatly needed specialty treatment.

Intensive Single-family and Multifamily Format

A short-term intensive family therapy (IFT), molded from FBT, has been tested across sites.[36,37] In IFT, families engage in a 5-day, 8-h/d treatment week; this intensive format may be a particularly helpful alternative for families who cannot regularly access specialty ED care, and may also serve as an option for treatment-resistant cases.[38] A multifamily therapy approach to ED treatment was developed with the hypothesis that it would hold some benefits compared with the single-family format.[39] Specifically, a multiple-family format is predicated on the supposition that, when bringing families together as groups, family resources and support for one another are amplified, which may then lead to improved outcomes.[40] Prospective study of IFT in both single-family IFT (S-IFT) and multifamily IFT (M-IFT) formats was conducted with 74 adolescents.[36] Full remission was defined as normal weight ($\geq$95% of expected for sex, age, and height), EDE Questionnaire (EDE-Q) global scores within 1 SD of norms, and absence of binge-purge behaviors. Partial remission was defined as weight greater than or equal to 85% of expected or greater than or equal to 95% but with increased EDE-Q global score and presence of binge-purging symptoms (<1 per week). Over a mean follow-up of 30 months, results showed that 87.8% of participants achieved full (60.8%) or partial remission (27%), whereas 12.2% reported a poor outcome. Notably, findings indicated that both formats had comparable outcomes in achieving full or partial remission. Taken together, preliminary evidence suggests that short-term, intensive treatments, in both S-IFT and M-IFT formats, may confer overall positive treatment outcomes. These findings confirm that a multiple-family treatment format is no less effective, and may serve to improve accessibility, increase use of mutual family support, and provide a higher level of care that is less disruptive.

Family-based Treatment of Transition-aged Youth

Most of the extant FBT literature has focused on adolescents between the ages of 12 and 18 years. However, the definition of adolescence is mutable, and, particularly in Western societies, adolescence frequently extends into young adulthood. Transition-aged youth (TAY) (17–25 years old) are distinct from both adolescents and older adults because many continue to reside with family from whom they may receive substantial financial and emotional support, suggesting that adapting FBT for this patient population may be propitious.[41] In the context of EDs, previous research indicates that FBT might be less effective for older than for younger adolescents with AN,[40] but a recent feasibility and acceptability study for young adults found that FBT, with appropriate modifications, was able to achieve weight restoration in this patient population.[42] A manualized FBT-TAY builds on the model of FBT for adolescents with AN and BN, and incorporates adaptations that are appropriate for the developmental needs of older teenagers and young adults. These modifications include asking the young adults to describe what kind of support they need from family during mealtimes, thereby allowing them a say in how their treatment is delivered. Other modifications include considering developmentally appropriate situations (eg, eating on campus) and how recovery may include age-appropriate transition issues (eg, return to work, living with a partner or friends). In a recent small trial of FBT-TAY with 26 participants, findings indicated significant improvement in EDE-Q global scores at end of treatment and 3 months posttreatment.[43,44] Participants also achieved and maintained weight restoration at end of treatment and 3 months posttreatment compared with baseline, suggesting that FBT-TAY is a promising adaptation of FBT for which a larger clinical trial is warranted.

Family-based Treatment of Other Eating and Weight Disorders

To date, clinical trials in ED diagnoses other than AN and BN are limited, and no clinical trials have specifically examined FBT for binge-eating disorder. Recognizing that obesity in youth is a public health concern and has a predictable course of obesity into adulthood, FBT for pediatric obesity (FBT-PO) has been proposed, with preliminary testing in a case study and RCT.[45,46] In FBT-PO, the treatment approach is modified according to the age of the patient. Parents are involved at the beginning of treatment to varying degrees, depending on the maturity of the child and not the severity of the "illness," to account for the absence of interfering mental disorders. Parents initially assume full responsibility for eating-related and exercise-related changes in the home, and all family-level modifications are health oriented, safe, and applicable even for nonoverweight family members. As with FBT-AN, parental control over eating and exercise lessens over the course of treatment.

Several research groups are developing and investigating versions of FBT for avoidant resistant food intake disorder (ARFID) (eg, Ref.[47]). In an FBT model currently being adapted for ARFID, psychoeducation is provided about features unique to this disorder. The focus of treatment is on empowering parents, restoring weight as necessary, uniting the family against the ED, and improving eating behaviors to include a greater variety of foods. As research continues to improve understanding of ED diagnoses clarified by DSM-5, adapting FBT treatments for suitable use in these populations implicates promising avenues to address a wider array of ED symptoms in a greater variety of formats and forums.

ADAPTATIONS OF FAMILY-BASED TREATMENTS BASED ON TREATMENT OUTCOME MODERATORS

Evidence from studies of moderators that may affect treatment outcomes in RCTs for FBT-AN and FBT-BN has guided specific adaptations in treatment protocols. Specifically, early weight gain,[48] parental criticism,[49] and obsessionality[24] have all been identified as moderators that may significantly and negatively affect FBT treatment outcomes. To address each of these moderators in turn, modified versions of FBT have been tested.

Early weight gain (a specific degree of weight gain by 1 month of manualized FBT) is a strong early predictor of remission.[24,25,48,50] Parental self-efficacy is a proven mediator of FBT treatment outcomes, suggesting that maneuvering weight gain early in treatment may assist parents in becoming more empowered within the context of FBT, thereby improving overall weight gain at end of treatment.[51] For those adolescents with AN who are considered nonresponders in not gaining a sufficient amount of weight (2.4 kg) in the first month of manualized FBT treatment, an adaptive treatment approach, with intensive parental coaching (IPC), has been developed. In this treatment augmentation protocol, sessions 4 through 6 follow a specific format with the intent to enhance parental self-efficacy in families of early nonresponders. Specifically, session 4 introduces the adaptive treatment, and reemphasizes the importance of weight gain. Parents receive a session alone (ie, session 5 is a separated family session) to orchestrate a renewed intense scene about the severity of illness, and reinvigorate a sense of immediacy in the need for weight restoration. In addition, in session 6, parents participate with their adolescent in a second family meal. In one study of this adaptive treatment, 45 adolescents with AN were randomized to either FBT (n = 10) or FBT with IPC (n = 35) if patients did not gain 2.4 kg by session 4. In addition to standard FBT, IPC included 3 additional sessions (ie, sessions 4–6). At end of treatment, patients receiving FBT-IPC had gained significantly more weight than patients continuing after session 4 with standard FBT.[27] Results should be interpreted with caution given the small sample size, but preliminary results suggest that this adaptive FBT may be effective in ultimately eliciting weight restoration for early treatment nonresponders. A confirmatory multisite trial of this adaptive treatment is currently being conducted with a 2-site sample of adolescents with AN and their families.

Several studies have shown that parental criticism, as measured by expressed emotion, can negatively affect treatment outcomes.[41,49,52] To address this issue, a recent RCT compared FBT with PFT, a separated version of the same treatment.[26,53] In PFT, the adolescent is seen at the beginning of the session and weighed, with brief supportive counseling. The remainder of the session is spent meeting alone with the parents. In this study of 107 adolescents with AN comparing conjoint FBT with the separated format (PFT), remission rates were higher in PFT (43%) than in FBT (22%) at end of treatment. However, the treatment groups did not differ at 6-month or 12-month follow-up.[26] Regardless of remission rates, reduction in criticism is much more likely to occur within the context of PFT, rather than FBT. These findings provide preliminary evidence that PFT can be an effective treatment of adolescents with AN, and perhaps preferred for families with baseline parental criticism.

When individuals present with greater severity in perseverative ED thinking or obsessive-compulsive features, FBT is superior to AFT in achieving weight restoration.[41] This finding suggests that a more behavioral approach, such as FBT, is better equipped to address this mental disorder than an individual psychotherapy. However, individuals with this cognitive presentation may require a longer course of FBT.[24] Relatedly, preliminary research suggests that cognitive remediation therapy (CRT) is feasible and acceptable to adolescents with AN, and could reduce the effects on cognitive inflexibility on treatment outcome, as indicated in recent work.[54] Thirty adolescents meeting criteria for DSM-5 diagnosis of AN, who also reported perseverative thinking, were randomized to manualized FBT plus CRT, or manualized FBT plus art therapy. because both groups gained weight and showed improvements on the EDE, it remains unclear whether adding a targeted and specific individual therapy to FBT aimed at perseverative thinking is worthy of further study.

Treatment adaptations that have targeted early weight gain, parental criticism, and cognitive rigidity show promise in improving precision treatment efforts in specific populations. Continued study of predictors of response to FBT in both AN and BN and the factors that moderate the effects of treatment on outcome are critical to the development of more precise and tailored treatment efforts. This study is particularly needed for BN, for which moderators of outcome have been less studied.

FUTURE DIRECTIONS

Systematic review of AN treatment across both adolescents and adults indicates that specialty treatments, including FBT, are more adept than comparator interventions at achieving weight-based improvement at end of treatment, but that psychological symptom relief does not follow a commensurate course.[55] Within FBT for adolescents specifically, weight restoration is an explicit focus; based on evidence that early weight gain in the context of treatment is critical (eg, Ref.[25]), future study of FBT adaptations that increase early weight gain may improve indices of weight restoration at follow-up. To address the latency of psychological symptoms in the context of recovery, improving the implementation of FBT across specific populations for whom standard FBT is less effective may greatly improve treatment response.

Perhaps even more important than improving the efficacy of FBT is increasing its dissemination capacity. Access to specialty providers for ED treatment is a challenge outside of urban environs, and there are a limited number of trained providers outside the specific sites where FBT was developed.[56] Increasing access to FBT training through Web-based education and supervision is a key area of development. In addition, preliminary effectiveness for the delivery of FBT via telehealth has been established[34,35] and warrants further examination across a larger trial. A recent examination of a parental guided self-help format of treatment of adolescents with AN showed initial feasibility and may also serve to extend treatment services beyond what is available with in-person providers.[57]

SUMMARY AND DISCUSSION

The last decade has witnessed advances in the development of FBT for adolescent EDs, particularly in the study of AN but also with a recent, notable initiation in study of FBT for BN. Taken together, there is a robust body of evidence supporting the efficacy of interventions that emphasize family involvement. Further research is needed to investigate the precise nature of optimal family involvement, and specifically to determine for whom, and under what conditions, certain types of family involvement might be most effective. In addition, the dissemination of specialty treatments such as FBT is crucial to the advancement of precision medical treatment of ED in adolescents, toward which concerted efforts should be directed.

REFERENCES

1. Steinhausen HC. The outcome of anorexia nervosa in the 20th century. Am J Psychiatry 2002;159(8):1284–93.
2. Swanson SA, Crow SJ, Le Grange D, et al. Prevalence and correlates of eating disorders in adolescents: results from the national comorbidity survey replication adolescent supplement. Arch Gen Psychiatry 2011;68(7):714–23.
3. Anastasiadou D, Medina-Pradas C, Sepulveda AR, et al. A systematic review of family caregiving in eating disorders. Eat Behav 2014;15(3):464–77.
4. Agras WS. The consequences and costs of the eating disorders. Psychiatr Clin North Am 2001;24(2):371–9.
5. Treasure J, Russell G. The case for early intervention in anorexia nervosa: theoretical exploration of maintaining factors. Br J Psychiatry 2011;199(1):5–7.
6. Lock J, Le Grange D. Family-based treatment: where are we and where should we be going to improve recovery in child and adolescent eating disorders. Int J Eat Disord 2018. [Epub ahead of print].
7. National Institute for Health and Care Excellence. Eating disorders: recognition and treatment (NICE guideline NH69) 2017. Available at: https://www.nice.org.uk/guidance/ng69. Accessed May 23, 2017.
8. Hilbert A, Hoek HW, Schmidt R. Evidence-based clinical guidelines for eating disorders: international comparison. Curr Opin Psychiatry 2017;30(6):423.
9. Le Grange D, Lock J. The dearth of psychological treatment studies for anorexia nervosa. Int J Eat Disord 2005;37:79–91.
10. Hail L, Le Grange D. Bulimia nervosa in adolescents: prevalence and treatment challenges. Adolesc Health Med Ther 2018;9:11.
11. Loeb KL, Le Grange D, Lock J. Family therapy for adolescent eating and weight disorders: new applications. 1st edition. New York: Routledge/Taylor and Francis Group; 2015.
12. Stiles-Shields C, Rienecke Hoste RM, Doyle P, et al. A review of family-based treatment for adolescents with eating disorders. Rev Recent Clin Trials 2012; 7(2):133–40.
13. Le Grange D, Eisler I. Family interventions in adolescent anorexia nervosa. Child Adolesc Psychiatr Clin N Am 2009;18(1):159–73.
14. Le Grange D, Lock J, Loeb K, et al. Academy for eating disorders position paper: the role of the family in eating disorders. Int J Eat Disord 2010;43(1):1–5.
15. Schmidt U, Treasure J. Anorexia nervosa: valued and visible. A cognitive-interpersonal maintenance model and its implications for research and practice. Br J Clin Psychol 2006;45(3):343–66.
16. Le Grange D, Lock J. Treating bulimia in adolescents: a family-based approach. Guilford Press; 2009.
17. Eisler I. The empirical and theoretical base of family therapy and multiple family day therapy for adolescent anorexia nervosa. J Fam Ther 2005;27(2):104–31.
18. Russell GF, Szmukler GI, Dare C, et al. An evaluation of family therapy in anorexia nervosa and bulimia nervosa. Arch Gen Psychiatry 1987;44(12):1047–56.
19. Lock J, Le Grange D. Treatment manual for anorexia nervosa: a family-based approach. 2nd Edition. New York: Guilford Publications; 2013.
20. Le Grange D, Lock J. Treating bulimia in adolescents: a family-based approach. Guilford Press; 2007.

21. Lock J, Le Grange D, Agras WS, et al. Randomized clinical trial comparing family-based treatment with adolescent-focused individual therapy for adolescents with anorexia nervosa. Arch Gen Psychiatry 2010;67(10):1025–32.

22. Fairburn CG, Cooper I. The eating disorder examination. In: Fairburn CG, Wilson GT, editors. Binge eating: nature, assessment, and treatment. 12th edition. New York: Guilford Press; 1993.

23. Agras WS, Lock J, Brandt H, et al. Comparison of 2 family therapies for adolescent anorexia nervosa: a randomized parallel trial. JAMA Psychiatry 2014;71(11):1279–86.

24. Lock J, Agras WS, Bryson S, et al. A comparison of short-and long-term family therapy for adolescent anorexia nervosa. J Am Acad Child Adolesc Psychiatry 2005;44(7):632–9.

25. Madden S, Miskovic-Wheatley J, Wallis A, et al. Early weight gain in family-based treatment predicts greater weight gain and remission at the end of treatment and remission at 12-month follow-up in adolescent anorexia nervosa. Int J Eat Disord 2015;48(7):919–22.

26. Le Grange D, Hughes EK, Court A, et al. Randomized clinical trial of parent-focused treatment and family-based treatment for adolescent anorexia nervosa. J Am Acad Child Adolesc Psychiatry 2016;55:683–92.

27. Lock J, Le Grange D, Agras WS, et al. Can adaptive treatment improve outcomes in family-based therapy for adolescents with anorexia nervosa? Feasibility and treatment effects of a multi-site treatment study. Behav Res Ther 2015;73:90–5.

28. Le Grange D, Loeb KL, Van Orman S, et al. Bulimia nervosa in adolescents: a disorder in evolution? Arch Pediatr Adolesc Med 2004;158(5):478–82.

29. Schmidt U, Lee S, Beecham J, et al. A randomized controlled trial of family therapy and cognitive behavior therapy guided self-care for adolescents with bulimia nervosa and related disorders. Am J Psychiatry 2007;164(4):591–8.

30. Fairburn CG, Marcus MD, Wilson GT. Cognitive-behavioral therapy for binge eating and bulimia nervosa: a comprehensive treatment manual. In: Fairburn CG, Wilson GT, editors. Binge eating: nature, assessment, and treatment. New York: Guilford Press; 1993. p. 361–404.

31. Le Grange D, Crosby RD, Rathouz PJ, et al. A randomized controlled comparison of family-based treatment and supportive psychotherapy for adolescent bulimia nervosa. Arch Gen Psychiatry 2007;64(9):1049–56.

32. Le Grange D, Lock J, Agras WS, et al. Randomized clinical trial of family-based treatment and cognitive-behavioral therapy for adolescent bulimia nervosa. J Am Acad Child Adolesc Psychiatry 2015;54(11):886–94.

33. Spieth PM, Kubasch AS, Penzlin AI, et al. Randomized controlled trials–a matter of design. Neuropsychiatr Dis Treat 2016;12:1341.

34. Anderson KE, Byrne C, Goodyear A, et al. Telemedicine of family-based treatment for adolescent anorexia nervosa: a protocol of a treatment development study. J Eat Disord 2015;3(1):25.

35. Anderson KE, Byrne CE, Crosby RD, et al. Utilizing Telehealth to deliver family-based treatment for adolescent anorexia nervosa. Int J Eat Disord 2017;50(10):1235–8.

36. Marzola E, Knatz S, Murray SB, et al. Short-term intensive family therapy for adolescent eating disorders: 30-month outcome. Eur Eat Disord Rev 2015;23(3):210–8.

37. Rockwell RE, Boutelle K, Trunko ME, et al. An innovative short-term, intensive, family-based treatment for adolescent anorexia nervosa: case series. Eur Eat Disord Rev 2011;19(4):362–7.

38. Knatz S, Kaye W, Marzola E, et al. A brief, intensive application of family based treatment for eating disorders. In: Loeb KL, Le Grange D, Lock J, editors. Family therapy for adolescent eating and weight disorders: new applications. New York: Routledge/Taylor and Francis Group; 2015. p. 72–91.

39. Simic M, Eisler I. Multi-family therapy. In: Loeb KL, Le Grange D, Lock J, editors. Family therapy for adolescent eating and weight disorders: new applications. New York: Routledge/Taylor and Francis Group; 2015. p. 110–38.

40. Eisler I, Simic M, Hodsoll J, et al. A pragmatic randomised multi-centre trial of multifamily and single family therapy for adolescent anorexia nervosa. BMC Psychiatry 2016;16(1):422.

41. Le Grange D, Lock J, Agras WS, et al. Moderators and mediators of remission in family-based treatment and adolescent focused therapy for anorexia nervosa. Behav Res Ther 2012;50(2):85–92.

42. Dimitropoulos G, Lock J, Le Grange D, et al. Family therapy for transition youth. In: Loeb KL, Le Grange D, Lock J, editors. Family therapy for adolescent eating and weight disorders: new applications. New York: Routledge/Taylor and Francis Group; 2015. p. 230–55.

43. Chen EY, Weissman JA, Zeffiro TA, et al. Family-based therapy for young adults with anorexia nervosa restores weight. Int J Eat Disord 2016;49(7):701–7.

44. Dimitropoulos G, Landers AL, Freeman V, et al. Open trial of family-based treatment of anorexia nervosa for transition age youth. J Can Acad Child Adolesc Psychiatry 2018;27(1):50.

45. Loeb KL, Celio Doyle A, Anderson K, et al. Family-based treatment for child and adolescent overweight and obesity: a transdevelopmental approach. In: Loeb KL, Le Grange D, Lock J, editors. Family therapy for adolescent eating and weight disorders: new applications. New York: Routledge; 2015. p. 177–229.

46. Stiles-Shields C, Doyle AC, Le Grange D, et al. J Contemp Psychother 2018. Available at: https://doi.org/10.1007/s10879-018-9399-6.

47. Fitzpatrick KK, Forsberg SE, Colborn D. Family-based therapy for avoidant restrictive food intake disorder: families facing food neophobias. In: Loeb KL, Le Grange D, Lock J, editors. Family therapy for adolescent eating and weight disorders: new applications. New York: Routledge/Taylor and Francis Group; 2015. p. 256–76.

48. Le Grange D, Accurso EC, Lock J, et al. Early weight gain predicts outcome in two treatments for adolescent anorexia nervosa. Int J Eat Disord 2014;47(2):124–9.

49. Eisler I, Dare C, Hodes M, et al. Family therapy for adolescent anorexia nervosa: the results of a controlled comparison of two family interventions. J Child Psychol Psychiatry 2000;41(6):727–36.

50. Doyle PM, Le Grange D, Loeb K, et al. Early response to family-based treatment for adolescent anorexia nervosa. Int J Eat Disord 2010;43(7):659–62.

51. Byrne CE, Accurso EC, Arnow KD, et al. An exploratory examination of patient and parental self-efficacy as predictors of weight gain in adolescents with anorexia nervosa. Int J Eat Disord 2015;48(7):883–8.

52. Allan E, Le Grange D, Sawyer SM, et al. Parental expressed emotion during two forms of family-based treatment for adolescent anorexia nervosa. Eur Eat Disord Rev 2018;26(1):46–52.

53. Hughes EK, Sawyer SM, Loeb KL, et al. Parent-focused treatment. In: Loeb KL, Le Grange D, Lock J, editors. Family therapy for adolescent eating and weight disorders: new applications. New York: Routledge/Taylor and Francis Group; 2015. p. 59–71.

54. Lock J, Fitzpatrick KK, Agras WS, et al. Feasibility study combining art therapy or cognitive remediation therapy with family-based treatment for adolescent anorexia nervosa. Eur Eat Disord Rev 2018;26(1):62–8.
55. Murray SB, Quintana DS, Loeb KL, et al. Treatment outcomes for anorexia nervosa: a systematic review and meta-analysis of randomized controlled trials. Psychol Med 2018;49(4):1–10.
56. Murray SB, Le Grange D. Family therapy for adolescent eating disorders: an update. Curr Psychiatry Rep 2014;16(5):447.
57. Lock J, Darcy A, Fitzpatrick KK, et al. Parental guided self-help family based treatment for adolescents with anorexia nervosa: a feasibility study. Int J Eat Disord 2017;50(9):1104–8.

Interpersonal Psychotherapy and the Treatment of Eating Disorders

Anna M. Karam, MA[a], Ellen E. Fitzsimmons-Craft, PhD[b],
Marian Tanofsky-Kraff, PhD[c], Denise E. Wilfley, PhD[d],*

KEYWORDS

- Interpersonal psychotherapy (IPT) • Psychotherapy • Eating disorders
- Bulimia nervosa • Binge-eating disorder • Obesity

KEY POINTS

- Interpersonal psychotherapy (IPT) for eating disorders is an evidence-based treatment of bulimia nervosa and binge-eating disorder.
- IPT is a focused intervention that links the interpersonal and social context to eating disorder onset and maintenance.
- Given that IPT is effective for a range of psychological problems and that it can be considered a best buy intervention, efforts to widely disseminate this treatment should be continued.
- Future work should continue to study IPT, evaluate treatment moderators and mediators, and further promote the dissemination and implementation of IPT in clinical settings.

Interpersonal psychotherapy (IPT) is a time-limited and empirically supported treatment that assumes human relationships and an individual's social and interpersonal context are central to mental health. IPT has been studied for decades, and numerous randomized controlled trials have provided strong support for its efficacy,[1] including

Disclosures statement: A.M. Karam, E.E. Fitzsimmons-Craft, and M. Tanofsky-Kraff have no conflicts of interest or commercial relationships related to this article to report. M. Tanofsky-Kraff provides the disclaimer that the opinions and assertions expressed herein are those of the authors and are not to be construed as reflecting the views of USUHS or the US Department of Defense. D.E. Wilfley has received an educational grant from Shire Pharmaceuticals to develop an interpersonal psychotherapy online training platform.

[a] Department of Psychology, Washington University in St. Louis, 660 South Euclid Avenue, Mailstop 8134-29-2100, St. Louis, MO 63110, USA; [b] Department of Psychiatry, Washington University School of Medicine, 660 South Euclid Avenue, Mailstop 8134-29-2100, St. Louis, MO 63110, USA; [c] Department of Medical and Clinical Psychology, Uniformed Services University of the Health Sciences (USUHS), 4301 Jones Bridge Road, Bethesda, MD 20814-4712, USA; [d] Scott Rudolph University, Washington University School of Medicine, 660 South Euclid Avenue, Mailstop 8134-29-2100, St. Louis, MO 63110, USA
* Corresponding author.
E-mail address: wilfleyd@wustl.edu

Psychiatr Clin N Am 42 (2019) 205–218
https://doi.org/10.1016/j.psc.2019.01.003
0193-953X/19/© 2019 Elsevier Inc. All rights reserved.

for bulimia nervosa (BN) and binge-eating disorder (BED). This article describes IPT for eating disorders (EDs), discusses its history and evolution, reviews the empirical evidence that supports IPT's classification as an evidence-based treatment, summarizes efforts to disseminate and increase implementation of IPT, and discusses future directions.

IPT was first developed by Klerman and colleagues[2] as a brief, focused outpatient treatment of patients with depression in a randomized clinical trial. IPT was originally based on the interpersonal theories of Sullivan, Bowlby, and Meyer, which suggest interpersonal functioning is crucial to psychological well-being and adjustment. Although IPT makes no suppositions about the etiology of psychiatric illnesses, IPT assumes the onset and maintenance of these disorders and response to treatment occur in a social and interpersonal context. As such, the fundamental aim of IPT is to identify and alter the interpersonal patterns in which the problem has been developed and maintained. IPT has since been adapted for the treatment of a range of clinical disorders,[1] but all adaptations of IPT maintain a similar treatment structure and share core treatment components, such as the focus on interpersonal problem areas.

INTERPERSONAL PSYCHOTHERAPY FOR EATING DISORDERS

IPT was initially adapted for EDs by Fairburn and colleagues[3] in a comparative trial of 3 treatments of BN. Since then, IPT has been evaluated in numerous randomized controlled trials for EDs and is classified as a strongly supported evidence-based treatment of BN and BED.[4,5]

IPT was adapted for EDs based on theoretic underpinnings of the interpersonal model of binge eating,[6] which was adapted from interpersonal theories for depression.[2] The interpersonal model of binge-eating proposes interpersonal problems or social disturbances cause low self-esteem, dysphoria, and other aversive mood states, which lead to binge eating and other ED symptoms as means of coping (**Fig. 1**). Engaging in ED behaviors can further intensify social difficulties, perpetuating the cycle. Several research studies have provided support for aspects of the interpersonal model of binge eating as well as for the model as a whole. Research has consistently demonstrated the association between interpersonal problems and EDs.[7,8] It is also well documented that negative affect reliably precedes binge eating.[9] Finally, studies have empirically evaluated and found support for the interpersonal model of binge eating in a variety of samples and in laboratory experiments.[10,11]

Treatment Structure and Features

IPT is a short-term, focused treatment that relates behavioral symptoms to interpersonal problems and generally lasts 6 to 20 sessions. It is characterized by 3 phases (**Box 1** has an overview of IPT), each of which is associated with tasks and strategies

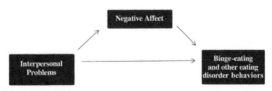

Fig. 1. The interpersonal model of binge eating.

Box 1
Outline of interpersonal psychotherapy

Initial phase
- Assess symptom presentation.
- Provide formal diagnosis and psychoeducation.
- Instill hope for the recovery process.
- Establish rapport.
- Conduct the interpersonal inventory.
- Develop the interpersonal case formulation.
  - Assign problem area(s).
  - Collaboratively develop treatment goals.

Intermediate phase
- Assess symptoms weekly.
- Relate symptoms to identified IPT problem area(s).
- Recognize connection between reduction in ED symptoms and improvements in interpersonal functioning.
- Implement IPT treatment strategies and tasks.
- Maintain focus on identified IPT treatment goals.

Termination phase
- Review progress.
- Outline remaining work.
- Discuss warning signs and relapse prevention.

---

that aim to identify and resolve a specified interpersonal problem area, including grief, interpersonal role disputes, role transitions, and/or interpersonal deficits (see Markowitz and Weissman[1] for more information on IPT).

Initial phase

The initial phase (sessions 1–5) is devoted to a comprehensive evaluation of a patient's interpersonal and symptom history. First, the patient's current and past symptoms are assessed. The therapist provides the patient with a formal diagnosis and psychoeducation about the disorder (eg, prevalence rates, clinical characteristics, and illness course) with the hope of removing blame from the patient and normalizing the problem. Expectations for treatment and the rationale for IPT are discussed, and the therapist instills hope and positive expectations for recovery by informing the patient of IPT's established efficacy. To determine the focus of treatment, the therapist conducts an interpersonal inventory, which aids in identifying the interpersonal problem area(s) connected to the onset and maintenance of ED symptoms and is then used to develop the interpersonal case formulation (both described in more detail later). IPT promotes a collaborative partnership between therapist and patient throughout the therapy course.

Problem areas The 4 problem areas addressed in IPT include grief, interpersonal role disputes, role transitions, and/or interpersonal deficits. Each problem area is described in **Table 1**. Typically, a single problem area is assigned as the focus of treatment, although it is possible that a patient may have more than 1 problem area.

Interpersonal inventory The interpersonal inventory links interpersonal events and the social context to ann illness timeline. The timeline helps therapists identify and label interpersonal patterns that emerge. It is considered an essential component of IPT

Table 1
Interpersonal problem areas ani Interpersonal psychotherapy treatment goals

Problem Area	Description	Interpersonal Psychotherapy Goals and Strategies
Grief	Death of a loved one that results in complicated bereavement	• Review sequence of events leading up to, during, and after death. • Facilitate the patient's mourning process. • Reconstruct the patient's relationship with the deceased. • Explore associated feelings, both negative and positive. • Re-establish interest in other relationships to substitute for what has been lost.
Interpersonal role disputes	Conflict(s) with a significant person (eg, partner, family member, close friend, or coworker)	• Identify the nature of the dispute. • Highlight how nonreciprocal role expectations relate to dispute. • Determine stage of dispute: renegotiation, i.mpasse, or dissolution. • Choose a plan of action • Identify available resources to bring about change in the relationship. • Modify expectations and faulty communication to bring about asatisfactory resolution.
Role transitions	Difficulty during a significant life change (eg, becoming a parent, beginning college, children leaving the home, job change, divorce, or retirement)	• Review positive and negative aspects of old and new roles. • Explore feelings about what is lost, emotions about the change itself, and opportunities in the new role. • Encourage development of social support system and new skills called for in new role.
Interpersonal deficits	A long-standing history of social impoverishment, isolation, unrewarding relationships, and/or an inability to form or maintain intimate relationships	• Review past significant relationships, including positive and negative aspects. • Explore repetitive patterns in relationships. • Encourage the formation of new relationships. • Reduce the patient's social isolation • Enhance quality of existing relationships.

Adapted from Burke NL, Karam AM, Tanofsky-Kraff M, et al. Interpersonal psychotherapy for the treatment of eating disorders. In: Agras WS, Robinson A, editors. The oxford handbook of eating disorders, 2nd edition. New York: Oxford University Press; 2018; with permission.

and is critical to the success of treatment. The interpersonal inventory involves the following:

- Providing a detailed and comprehensive review of the patient's
  - Important relationships currently and since illness onset

Therapists can assess past and present significant relationships by asking questions, such as

"Tell me about the people with whom you are closest to and confide in right now?"

"Tell me about the important people in your life when you first started having these symptoms?"

- ○ Interpersonal functioning currently and since illness onset
- ○ Social and interpersonal areas the therapist may probe about include family, school, military, confiding relationships, and romantic and sexual relationships; individuals the patient is in daily contact with; family of origin; friends and social supports; conflicted relationships; recent deaths; emotional losses; and changes in vocational status, health, and/or housing.

Therapists can assess present problems by asking questions, such as

"Tell me about a recent episode of binge eating. What was going on in your social environment and interpersonal relationships?"

Therapists can assess past symptoms and interpersonal functioning by asking questions, such as

"When was the first time you recall [feeling like this] [having behaviors like this]? How old were you?"

"What else was going on in your life at that time? For example, how were things at home? What were things like at school?.."

And "when" was the next period of time you [felt like this] [engaged in those behaviors]? "What" was going on socially for you then?

- • Illuminates interpersonal precipitants of illness episodes
- • Allows the therapist to make connections between the social and interpersonal context to symptoms

Interpersonal case formulation The interpersonal case formulation is customized to a patient's individualized history, synthesizes the initial phase of treatment, and sets the stage for the remaining treatment course. The formulation summarizes the interpersonal inventory and relates illness onset and maintenance to the problem area(s), and treatment goals are decided on collaboratively between therapist and patient. The problem area a patient is classified into is central to determining IPT treatment goals. **Table 1** delineates examples of common treatment strategies and goals for the 4 problem areas. The therapist explicitly verbalizes a summary of the interpersonal case formulation (including interpersonal pattern of symptoms, problem area[s], and treatment goals), and this should be negotiated until agreed on by both patient and therapist. The formulation is used as a transparent treatment strategy to aid in the transition from the initial phase to intermediate phase.

Intermediate phase
The intermediate phase (approximately 8–10 sessions) involves weekly assessment of symptoms and continually relating ED behaviors (or changes in such behaviors) to current interpersonal situations and events. A primary role of the therapist in the intermediate phase is to keep the patient focused on the problem area(s) and working toward the established goals. In doing so, the therapist inquires about treatment goals in each

intermediate session (eg, "How have you worked on your goals since we last met?"). There are several general therapeutic techniques used in IPT that work toward the established goals and are described in **Table 2**.

Termination phase

The termination phase (2–5 sessions) should be discussed explicitly with clients. Patients are educated about the end of treatment as a potential time for grieving; therapists should encourage patients to identify emotions associated with termination. During this phase, therapists also review client progress to foster feelings of accomplishment and competence, outline goals, and make specific plans for continued work after termination of treatment. Patients are informed of the importance of continued work in the interpersonal arena even after formal end of treatment to

Table 2
General therapeutic tasks and techniques used in the intermediate phase of interpersonal psychotherapy

Technique	Description
Exploration and clarification	• Therapist facilitates discussion of treatment-relevant information using general, open-ended questions often. • Therapist gains clarification by progressively following up with more specific questioning. • Clarification can help enhance patient's awareness to contradictions, which can occur through expressed or nonverbal (eg, showing a smile when describing being angry with significant other).
Therapeutic stance	• Therapist fosters positive therapeutic alliance through an attitude of warmth support and empathy. • Therapist is active, serves as patient advocate, and conveys an optimistic attitude about the patient's recovery. • Therapist focuses on current problems.
Focusing on goals	• Therapist keeps the patient focused on the problem areas and established goals throughout therapy course.
Redirect focus on symptoms	• Therapist redirects client focus on discussing symptoms to how symptoms are related to interpersonal problems.
Encourage affect	• Encourage acceptance of painful affect and to experience suppressed emotions. • Teach the patient how to use affect in interpersonal relationships. • Highlight emotional ambivalence. • Provide validation and reassurance.
Communication analysis	• Therapist collects detailed account of conversation or argument with significant other. • Explore feelings and intentions associated with communication. • Attend to nonreciprocal role expectations. • Watch for acts of commission or omission (eg, ambiguous, indirect, or nonverbal communication). • Assist patient with direct expression and appropriate assertion. • Discuss how the patient can plan for next conversation. • Role-plays are often used to practice communication skills.
Use of therapeutic relationship	• The therapist relationship can be used as an example of other relationships. • Discuss patient's positive and negative feelings about therapist and seek parallels in other relationships. • This strategy allows the therapist to identify problematic interpersonal processes that can be targeted during treatment.

maintain treatment gains and continue symptom improvement. Warning signs of relapse and anticipated future difficulty are identified and problem solved. Patients are reminded that interpersonal distress is sometimes associated with the re-emergence of ED symptoms and are encouraged to view such symptoms as early warning signals.

REVIEW OF RELEVANT EMPIRICAL LITERATURE
Interpersonal Psychotherapy for Bulimia Nervosa

Several studies have examined IPT's efficacy in the treatment of BN and have often compared IPT to cognitive behavior therapy (CBT).[3,12–15] Fairburn and colleagues[3] found that although both IPT and CBT produced significant improvement in BN psychopathology, CBT was superior to IPT in decreasing body weight and shape disturbances, extreme dieting behaviors, and self-induced vomiting at end of treatment. By 1-year and 6-year follow-ups, however, IPT and CBT produced similar, substantial improvements across symptomatology.[15] These results, which have also been confirmed by subsequent research, suggest that IPT catches up to CBT in terms of treatment efficacy and that both treatments have durable, long-lasting effects.[12,15] More recently, Fairburn and colleagues[16] compared CBT with IPT using a transdiagnostic ED sample (excluding anorexia nervosa [AN]). CBT produced superior end-of-treatment and 60-week follow-up remission rates compared with IPT; however, over the follow-up period, the proportion of participants who met criteria for remission increased and especially so for those who received IPT.

Although clinical trials have shown that IPT for BN achieves symptom reduction effects at a slower rate compared with CBT, 1 potential reason for these attenuated effects could be due to failing to discuss ED symptoms and linking them to the interpersonal context or by removing IPT techniques that overlap with CBT.[13] IPT for BN remains the leading strongly supported evidence-based alternative to CBT for BN.[4,5]

Interpersonal Psychotherapy for Binge-eating Disorder

Wilfley and colleagues[17] evaluated the efficacy of group IPT versus group CBT for a sample of individuals with nonpurging BN (ie, BED). Unlike the control condition, those in the IPT and CBT groups demonstrated significant reductions in binge eating, with treatment gains maintained for both conditions at 6-month and 12-month follow-ups.[17] In a similar but larger trial,[18] both treatments produced comparable and substantial improvement in binge-eating recovery rates at end of treatment and 1-year follow-up. A more recent trial in patients with BED randomized to IPT, CBT-guided self-help, or behavioral weight loss showed no differences in ED symptomatology among the treatments at end of treatment.[19] By 2-year follow-up, however, IPT and CBT-guided self-help produced greater remission from binge eating compared with behavioral weight loss. This study also demonstrated IPT led to greater symptom improvement compared with the other treatments for those with low self-esteem and high ED psychopathology. In a study of the long-term efficacy of psychological treatments for BED 4 years after Wilfley and colleagues'[18] trial, Hilbert and colleagues[20] documented that both IPT and CBT produced substantial long-term recovery, partial remission, and clinically significant improvement in associated psychopathology. Although the treatments did not significantly differ at any time point, those who received IPT showed improvement in ED symptoms over the follow-up period, whereas those in the CBT group tended to show a worsening of symptoms. In summary, several trials have examined IPT in the treatment of BED, and findings show a pattern of substantial success in the short term and long term and demonstrate IPT is especially helpful for those with low self-esteem and high ED psychopathology.

Interpersonal Psychotherapy for Anorexia Nervosa

Currently no evidence-based treatment exists for adults with AN,[4,5] and there is a lack of research examining IPT utility in this disorder. One study randomized 56 adults with AN to IPT, CBT, or nonspecific supportive clinical management.[21] Findings indicated that of the 3 therapies, nonspecific supportive clinical management was the most effective approach in terms of reductions in AN diagnostic features. Important to consider is that the investigators theorized these findings may be the result of the relative lack of focus on making connections between the IPT problem area and symptoms.[21] In a long-term follow-up 6 years to 7 years later, all 3 treatment groups were similar in ED symptomatology, anthropometrics, and general psychopathology,[22] and those who received IPT improved the most, relatively, across the follow-up period. These findings suggest that IPT may be of some benefit to individuals with AN and, similar to IPT for BN and BED, some individuals continue to improve even after the end of treatment.

Given the importance of interpersonal functioning in etiologic theories of AN,[21] additional research on IPT for AN is needed. Due to the medical severity and complexity that often accompanies AN, IPT may be more appropriately delivered for those with AN in conjunction with other treatments (eg, nutritional, pharmacologic) rather than a stand-alone treatment or for maintenance and relapse prevention after weight restoration.[23]

Interpersonal Psychotherapy in Adolescents for Prevention of Excessive Weight Gain

IPT has been modified for the prevention of excessive weight gain in adolescents who report loss-of-control eating and are high risk for adult obesity due to body mass index (BMI) percentile.[24] Loss-of-control eating is predictive of excess body weight, increased psychological problems, and the development of clinical eating pathology, such as BED, later in life.[25] IPT for prevention of excessive weight gain maintains core components of traditional IPT, provides additional psychoeducation about risk factors for excessive weight gain, and teaches additional general skill-building (eg, exercises that instruct adolescents to "put yourself in their shoes [and communicate it to them]"; see Burke and colleagues[23] for descriptions of these skills). Pilot studies and randomized controlled trials comparing IPT for prevention of excessive weight gain and a standard health education program have provided some support for this adaptation of IPT.[26] A pilot trial demonstrated the treatment was both feasible and acceptable to adolescent girls, and IPT for preventing weight gain produced less than expected increases in BMI and greater reductions in loss-of-control eating episodes compared with girls in the control group.[24] A randomized controlled trial showed IPT for preventing weight gain was not markedly better than health education for BMI or adiposity at 1-year or 3-year follow-up,[27,28] although at 1-year follow-up, girls in IPT reported significantly fewer binge-eating episodes compared with the health education control. Providing additional support for IPT, at 3-year follow-up, girls with greater anxiety or social maladjustment at baseline had greater improvements in BMI if randomized to IPT, and only those with higher anxiety who received IPT did not gain fat over time. Thus, consistent with IPT theory, IPT for the prevention of excess weight gain may be best suited for those with high anxiety and social problems.[27] Finally, IPT may be particularly useful for older girls and individuals from ethnic minority backgrounds in terms of BMI gain and loss-of-control eating compared with controls.[28,29] IPT for preventing excess weight gain and EDs has been modified for use in adolescent girls and boys of military service members; this adaptation demonstrated feasibility in a pilot trial, and an adequately powered randomized controlled trial is under way.[23]

In summary, numerous studies have evaluated IPT for EDs, and findings demonstrate a strong pattern of efficacy after treatment and beyond.[30]

Predictors, Moderators, and Mediators of Interpersonal Psychotherapy for Eating Disorders

Predictors, moderators, and mediators of treatment outcome could improve understanding of how treatments produce their effects and for whom, or under what conditions, they work best.[31] In terms of IPT for BN, lower levels of ED psychopathology[14,32] and higher self-esteem[13,14,33] at baseline have been found to consistently predict a more favorable outcome. Given these findings, therapists should consider trying to foster self-esteem during treatment, particularly in the early stages. No consistent treatment moderators have been identified to date. Regarding mediators, early symptom improvement[34,35] and stronger therapeutic alliance[36,37] have been found to consistently mediate outcome in IPT for BN. Therapists should work to facilitate a rapid treatment response and establish a good therapeutic alliance.

In terms of IPT for BED, less severe ED psychopathology,[38] older age of onset,[39] and shorter illness duration[32] have been found to predict a more promising outcome. Given these findings, individuals with BED should seek IPT treatment as early as possible. As described previously, Wilson and colleagues[19] found ED psychopathology to be a moderator of outcome in that those with higher levels of pathology improved most in IPT. Self-esteem has been identified as a moderator of treatment outcome in 2 studies, although implications of these findings are mixed. One study demonstrated that those with lower self-esteem were more likely to abstain from binge eating at end of treatment if they received IPT compared with CBT-guided self-help or behavioral weight loss,[19] yet another study found patients with lower self-esteem performed better in a full-course CBT than IPT.[32] Although these findings are mixed, it seems individuals with BED with low self-esteem should seek a full course of treatment, such as IPT or CBT, instead of a lower level of care (eg, guided self-help). No consistent treatment mediators have yet been identified in studies of IPT for BED. In a theoretical article of how IPT achieves its transdiagnostic treatment effects, Lipsitz and Markowitz[40] propose IPT activates several change mechanisms, including enhancing social support, decreasing interpersonal stress, facilitating emotional processing, and improving interpersonal skills (**Fig. 2**).

DISSEMINATION AND IMPLEMENTATION OF INTERPERSONAL PSYCHOTHERAPY

IPT is considered a best buy intervention because it has shown promising effects in treating and preventing a wide range of psychological problems.[41] IPT is an evidence-based treatment of both depression and EDs and also has been shown helpful in treating anxiety disorders, posttraumatic stress disorder, and bipolar disorder, and it is recommended for treating and preventing depression in pregnant and postpartum women.[41,42] Outside of AN, a disorder for which no evidence-based treatment of adults exists, IPT is appropriate for nearly all ED presentations, including subclinical binge-type disorders.[23] Although studied to a lesser extent, IPT has demonstrated positive effects when delivered to cocaine abusers, breast cancer patients, prostate and breast cancer survivors, and those with major physical trauma, bipolar depression, insomnia, and myocardial infarction.[41] The best buy nature of IPT

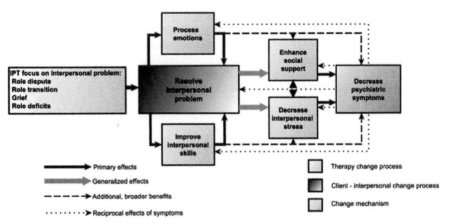

Fig. 2. Hypothesized interpersonal change processes and mechanisms in IPT. (*From* Lipsitz JD, Markowitz JC. Mechanisms of change in interpersonal therapy (IPT). Clin Psychol Rev 2013;33(8):1139; with permission.)

and its transdiagnostic flexibility to address a range of psychopathology make it particularly well suited for widespread dissemination and implementation efforts.[43]

Efforts to disseminate IPT to broader populations beyond those with EDs have shown promise. Stein and colleagues[44] compared 2 therapist training methods (ie, in-person training vs online training) for interpersonal and social rhythm therapy and found both training methods produced comparable rates of treatment uptake in practitioners. Additionally, the Veterans Health Administration conducted a national initiative for disseminating evidence-based treatments into their clinical care settings, including IPT for depression.[45] This training involved a 3-day workshop and 6 months of weekly telephone consultation with an IPT expert and showed promising results, including high scores of competence among therapists, and patients treated with IPT reported significant reductions in depressive symptoms and improvements in quality of life.[45] The widespread dissemination and implementation of this training initiative is suggestive of the feasibility and effectiveness of the broad dissemination of IPT to clinical care settings.

Initial efforts have also been made to evaluate the dissemination and implementation of IPT for EDs in clinical settings. For example, Wilfley and colleagues[46] have a project under way to examine the dissemination and implementation of IPT for EDs in college counseling centers across the United States in a National Institutes of Health–funded trial[46] (ClinicalTrials.gov identifier NCT02079142). This study is comparing the efficacy of 2 training models: (1) an in-person IPT training workshop with an expert with 12 months of follow-up consultation and (2) training a counseling center staff member in IPT who is then coached to train other staff members to implement IPT within their site (ie, a train-the-trainer model).

Another promising dissemination approach for IPT for EDs is online training because, in addition to being capable of training large numbers of therapists simultaneously, other potential advantages relative to traditional in-person training include increased cost-effectiveness, accessibility, and convenience.[43] Wilfley[47] is currently conducting a pilot trial to investigate an IPT online training program and telephone-based simulation assessment of therapist fidelity. The online training program and telephone-based simulation assessment are streamlined and scalable training and assessment resources. More scalable IPT training methods are needed and could enhance access to quality care and patient outcomes. Furthermore, for greater dissemination, implementation, and access to evidence-based care, higher-level support and policy efforts (eg, guidelines and systematic methods for organizing evidence-based treatment recommendations) are needed.[43]

FUTURE DIRECTIONS AND CONCLUSIONS

Several important areas of IPT for EDs require further study. To better understand the full range of problems that can be targeted using IPT, future research should continue to evaluate IPT for AN and IPT for excessive weight gain as well as IPT for other psychological problems. With the goal of continually enhancing IPT for EDs and increasing its utility, additional research also should be devoted to evaluating this treatment in understudied populations (eg, IPT for adolescents with EDs) and better understanding moderators and mediators of IPT in disorders for which it is known to be highly effective (ie, BN and BED), because more knowledge of treatment moderators provides insight into for whom or under which conditions IPT is most effective. Furthermore, identifying mediators of IPT would increase mechanistic understanding of how IPT achieves its therapeutic effects, and future treatment research could enhance the active therapeutic components (ie, treatment mediators), which could lead to the development of a more potent IPT.[29] Knowledge of disorders IPT effectively treats, whom IPT works most effectively for, and how IPT produces its effects is only useful insofar as therapists have access to IPT training and implement this treatment in clinical care settings with patients. Thus, another important future direction is additional work in the area of dissemination and implementation of IPT so that it is readily accessible for therapists to learn and patients to receive.

In conclusion, IPT is a time-limited, evidence-based treatment that assumes the development and maintenance of ED symptoms occur within a social and interpersonal context. IPT helps patients reduce symptoms by improving social functioning, repairing and building supports, improving communication, and resolving interpersonal problems. IPT consistently produces significant and well-maintained improvements in the treatment of BN and BED, and preliminary research supports IPT for the prevention of excess weight gain in adolescent girls. Additional research is needed to determine the effectiveness of IPT for AN. Finally, important future directions include additional research on IPT for other psychological problems, moderators and mediators of IPT for EDs, and more efforts that target the dissemination and implementation of IPT.

REFERENCES

1. Markowitz JC, Weissman MM. Casebook of interpersonal psychotherapy. New York: Oxford University Press; 2012.
2. Klerman GL, Weissman MM, Rounsaville BJ, et al. Interpersonal psychotherapy of depression. New York: Basic Books; 1984.
3. Fairburn CG, Jones R, Peveler RC, et al. Three psychological treatments for bulimia nervosa: A comparative trial. Arch Gen Psychiatry 1991;48(5):463–9.
4. APA Presidential Task Force on Evidence-Based Practice. Evidence-based practice in psychology. Am Psychol 2006;61:271–85.
5. Chambless DL, Hollon SD. Defining empirically supported therapies. J Consult Clin Psychol 1998;66(1):7.
6. Wilfley DE, MacKenzie RK, Welch RR, et al. Interpersonal psychotherapy for group. New York: Basic Books; 2000.

7. Arcelus J, Haslam M, Farrow C, et al. The role of interpersonal functioning in the maintenance of eating psychopathology: a systematic review and testable model. Clin Psychol Rev 2013;33(1):156–67.

8. Blomquist KK, Ansell EB, White MA, et al. Interpersonal problems and developmental trajectories of binge eating disorder. Compr Psychiatry 2012;53(8): 1088–95.

9. Berg KC, Cao L, Crosby RD, et al. Negative affect and binge eating: reconciling differences between two analytic approaches in ecological momentary assessment research. Int J Eat Disord 2017;50(10):1222–30.

10. Ivanova IV, Tasca GA, Proulx G, et al. Does the interpersonal model apply across eating disorder diagnostic groups? A structural equation modeling approach. Compr Psychiatry 2015;63:80–7.

11. Shank LM, Crosby RD, Grammer AC, et al. Examination of the interpersonal model of loss of control eating in the laboratory. Compr Psychiatry 2017;76: 36–44.

12. Agras WS, Walsh BT, Fairburn CG, et al. A multicenter comparison of cognitive-behavioral therapy and interpersonal psychotherapy for bulimia nervosa. Arch Gen Psychiatry 2000;57:459–66.

13. Arcelus J, Whight D, Langham C, et al. A case series evaluation of a modified version of interpersonal psychotherapy (IPT) for the treatment of bulimic eating disorders: a pilot study. Eur Eat Disord Rev 2009;17(4):260–8.

14. Fairburn CG, Peveler RC, Jones R, et al. Predictors of 12-month outcome in bulimia nervosa and the influence of attitudes to shape and weight. J Consult Clin Psychol 1993;61(4):696.

15. Fairburn CG, Norman PA, Welch SL, et al. A prospective study of outcome in bulimia nervosa and the long-term effects of three psychological treatments. Arch Gen Psychiatry 1995;52(4):304–12.

16. Fairburn CG, Bailey-Straebler S, Basden S, et al. A transdiagnostic comparison of enhanced cognitive behavior therapy (CBT-E) and interpersonal psychotherapy in the treatment of eating disorders. Behav Res Ther 2015;70:64–71.

17. Wilfley DE, Agras WS, Rossiter, et al. Group cognitive-behavioral therapy and group interpersonal psychotherapy for the nonpurging bulimic individual: a controlled comparison. J Consult Clin Psychol 1993;61(2):296.

18. Wilfley DE, Welch RR, Stein RI, et al. A randomized comparison of group cognitive-behavioral therapy and group interpersonal psychotherapy for the treatment of overweight individuals with binge-eating disorder. Arch Gen Psychiatry 2002;59(8):713–21.

19. Wilson GT, Wilfley DE, Agras WS, et al. Psychological treatments of binge eating disorder. Arch Gen Psychiatry 2010;67(1):94–101.

20. Hilbert A, Bishop ME, Stein RI, et al. Long-term efficacy of psychological treatments for binge eating disorder. Br J Psychiatry 2012;200(3):232–7.

21. McIntosh VV, Jordan J, Carter FA, et al. Three psychotherapies for anorexia nervosa: a randomized, controlled trial. Am J Psychiatry 2005;162(4):741–7.

22. Carter FA, Jordan J, McIntosh VVW. The long-term efficacy of three psychotherapies for anorexia nervosa: a randomized, controlled trial. Int J Eat Disord 2011; 44(7):647–54.

23. Burke NL, Karam AM, Tanofsky-Kraff M, et al. The Oxford handbook of eating disorders. In: Agras WS, Robinson A, editors. Interpersonal psychotherapy for the treatment of eating disorders. New York: Oxford University Press; 2017. p. 287–318.

24. Tanofsky-Kraff M, Wilfley DE, Young JF, et al. A pilot study of interpersonal psychotherapy for preventing excess weight gain in adolescent girls at-risk for obesity. Int J Eat Disord 2010;43(8):701–6.
25. Tanofsky-Kraff M, Yanovski SZ, Schvey NA, et al. A prospective study of loss of control eating for body weight gain in children at high risk for adult obesity. Int J Eat Disord 2009;42:26–30.
26. Shomaker LB, Tanofsky-Kraff M, Matherne CE, et al. A randomized, comparative pilot trial of family-based interpersonal psychotherapy for reducing psychosocial symptoms, disordered eating, and excess weight gain in at-risk preadolescents with loss-of-control-eating. Int J Eat Disord 2017;50(9):1084–94.
27. Tanofsky-Kraff M, Shomaker LB, Wilfley DE, et al. Excess weight gain prevention in adolescents: Three-year outcome following a randomized-controlled trial. J Consult Clin Psychol 2017;85(3):218–27.
28. Burke NL, Shomaker LB, Brady S. Impact of age and race on outcomes of a program to prevent excess weight gain and disordered eating in adolescent girls. Nutrients 2017;9(9):947.
29. Tanofsky-Kraff M, Shomaker LB, Wilfley DE, et al. Targeted prevention of excess weight gain and eating disorders in high-risk adolescent girls: a randomized controlled trial. Am J Clin Nutr 2014;100(4):1010–8.
30. Miniati M, Callari A, Maglio A, et al. Interpersonal psychotherapy for eating disorders: current perspectives. Psychol Res Behav Manag 2018;11:353.
31. Kraemer HC, Wilson GT, Fairburn CG, et al. Mediators and moderators of treatment effects in randomized clinical trials. Arch Gen Psychiatry 2002;59(10): 877–83.
32. Cooper Z, Allen E, Bailey-Straebler S, et al. Predictors and moderators of response to enhanced cognitive behavior therapy and interpersonal psychotherapy for the treatment of eating disorders. Behav Res Ther 2016;84:9–13.
33. Fairburn CG, Kirk J, O'Connor M, et al. Prognostic factors in bulimia nervosa. Br J Clin Psychol 1987;26(3):233–4.
34. Fairburn CG, Agras WS, Walsh BT, et al. Prediction of outcome in bulimia nervosa by early change in treatment. Am J Psychiatry 2004;161(12):2322–4.
35. Wilson GT, Fairburn CC, Agras WS, et al. Cognitive-behavioral therapy for bulimia nervosa: time course and mechanisms of change. J Consult Clin Psychol 2002; 70(2):267.
36. Constantino MJ, Arnow BA, Blasey C, et al. The association between patient characteristics and the therapeutic alliance in cognitive-behavioral and interpersonal therapy for bulimia nervosa. J Consult Clin Psychol 2005;73(2):203.
37. Leob KL, Wilson GT, Labouvie E, et al. Therapeutic alliance and treatment adherence in two interventions for bulimia nervosa: a study of process and outcome. J Consult Clin Psychol 2005;73(6):1097.
38. Hilbert A, Saelen BE, Stein RI, et al. Pretreatment and process predictors of outcome in interpersonal and cognitive behavioral psychotherapy for binge eating disorder. J Consult Clin Psychol 2007;75(4):645.
39. Agras WS, Telch CF, Arnow B, et al. Does interpersonal therapy help patients with binge eating disorder who fail to respond to cognitive-behavioral therapy? J Consult Clin Psychol 1995;63(3):356–60.
40. Lipsitz JD, Markowitz JC. Mechanisms of change in interpersonal therapy (IPT). Clin Psychol Rev 2013;33(8):1134–47.
41. Cuijpers P, Donker T, Weissman MM, et al. Interpersonal psychotherapy for mental health problems: a comprehensive meta-analysis. Am J Psychiatry 2016;173(7):680–7.

42. Draft Recommendation Statement: Perinatal Depression: Preventive Interventions. U.S. Preventive Service Task Force Web site. 2018. Available at: https://www.uspreventiveservicestaskforce.org/Page/Document/draft-recommendation-statement/perinatal-depression-preventive-interventions. Accessed November 2018.
43. Kazdin AE, Fitzsimmons-Craft EE, Wilfley DE. Addressing critical gaps in the treatment of eating disorders. Int J Eat Disord 2017;50(3):170–89.
44. Stein BD, Celedonia KL, Swartz H, et al. Implementing a web-based intervention to train community clinicans in an evidence-based psychotherapy: a pilot study. Psychiatr Serv 2015;66(9):988–91.
45. Stewart MO, Raffa SD, Steele JL, et al. National dissemination of interpersonal psychotherapy for depression in veterans: therapist and patient-level outcomes. J Consult Clin Psychol 2014;82(6):1201.
46. Wilfley DE, Fitzsimmons-Craft EE, Eichen DM, et al. Training models for implementing evidence-based psychological treatment for college mental health: a cluster randomized trial study protocol. Contemp Clin Trials 2018;72:117–25.
47. Wilfley DE. Harnessing technology for training clinicians to deliver interpersonal psychotherapy (IPT). Paper presented at the National Eating Disorders Association Conference. San Diego, CA, October 3, 2015.

Emerging Psychological Treatments in Eating Disorders

Emily M. Pisetsky, PhD[a],*, Lauren M. Schaefer, PhD[b],
Stephen A. Wonderlich, PhD[b,c], Carol B. Peterson, PhD[a]

KEYWORDS

- Anorexia nervosa • Bulimia nervosa • Binge-eating disorder • Psychotherapy
- Mindfulness • Neuromodulation

KEY POINTS

- Dialectical-behavioral therapy has accumulating data to support efficacy in bulimia nervosa and binge eating disorder.
- A small but growing body of evidence suggested acceptance-based treatment may have promise as alternate treatment for eating disorders.
- Integrative Cognitive Affective Therapy has lead to meaningful improvements in symptoms of bulimia nervosa.
- Neurocognitive treatments and neuromodulation treatments target cognitive patterns, brain regions, and neural circuits with promising preliminary evidence in the treatment of eating disorders.

INTRODUCTION

Evidenced-based treatments for eating disorders (EDs) include cognitive-behavioral therapy (CBT) and interpersonal psychotherapy for bulimia nervosa (BN) and binge-eating disorder (BED), family-based treatment for adolescent anorexia nervosa (AN), with some evidence supporting CBT for adult AN.[1,2] However, research findings suggest a strong need for improvements in treatment retention and outcome. Over the past decade, there has been an increase in research aimed at identifying the mechanisms contributing to the development and maintenance of ED symptoms and behaviors that can be targeted in treatment. As a result, several existing psychological treatments originally developed to address other forms of mental illness have been adapted for use in the treatment of EDs, and newer models of ED maintenance have spurred the

Disclosure Statement: Drs S.A. Wonderlich and C.B. Peterson receive royalties from Guilford Press.
[a] Department of Psychiatry, University of Minnesota, F282/2A West, 2450 Riverside Avenue, Minneapolis, MN 55454, USA; [b] Sanford Center for Biobehavioral Research, 120 South Eighth Street, Fargo, ND 58103, USA; [c] University of North Dakota School of Medicine and Health Sciences, Grand Forks, ND, USA
* Corresponding author.
E-mail address: episetsk@umn.edu

Psychiatr Clin N Am 42 (2019) 219–229
https://doi.org/10.1016/j.psc.2019.01.005
0193-953X/19/© 2019 Elsevier Inc. All rights reserved.

development of novel treatment approaches. These treatments have expanded traditional cognitive and interpersonal psychotherapies to directly address emotion regulation. Further, an increased understanding of cognitive neuroscience has led to the development and application of neurocognitive and neuromodulation treatments.

DIALECTICAL BEHAVIOR THERAPY
Theoretic Model

Dialectical behavior therapy (DBT) was originally developed to treat borderline personality disorder (BPD) and chronically suicidal individuals.[3] The biosocial theory underlying DBT posits that BPD develops when an individual's biological temperament consists of an increased sensitivity to emotional stimuli as well as a slow return to baseline in the context of an emotionally invalidating environment.[3] Therefore, enhancing patients' ability to adaptively regulate affective responses is a significant focus of treatment. Notably, problems in emotion regulation, emotion identification, and emotion awareness have been observed in EDs, and ED behaviors have been hypothesized to serve an emotion regulation function.[4–7] Further, overeating and restriction appear to exacerbate an individual's vulnerability to emotion dysregulation. As a result of both theoretic and empirical support, DBT has been adapted for EDs with a focus on cultivating healthy emotion-regulation skills, a balanced approach to eating, and living a life worth living.[8]

Structure of the Treatment

Phases/stages
DBT generally consists of 4 structural elements: individual therapy, skills group, coaching calls, and consultation group for therapists. However, some adaptations of DBT for EDs only use a subset of these elements. Group sessions are largely didactic in nature and cover the skills of *mindfulness* (which is considered the "core" skill of DBT), *emotion regulation*, *distress tolerance*, and *interpersonal effectiveness*. Individual therapy seeks to assist patients in applying these skills to specific behavioral targets, which are addressed in order of priority. Target 1 includes life-threatening behaviors such as suicide and parasuicide. Target 2 includes therapy-interfering behaviors such as not completing diary cards, refusing to be weighed, and substance abuse. Target 3 includes quality-of-life–interfering behaviors such as restrictive eating, binge eating, and purging. ED behaviors may be moved to Target 1 if the behaviors are potentially life-threatening (eg, ipecac use). Coaching calls are used between sessions to facilitate skill use in challenging real-life situations. Therapist consultation groups serve to enhance protocol adherence and provide a context for nonjudgmental professional feedback.

Clinical targets/techniques
The primary goal of DBT for EDs is to eliminate maladaptive ED behaviors (eg, binge eating, purging), and to work toward building a more fulfilling life. DBT is a structured treatment that includes teaching the *core skills* and reviewing *diary cards*, which are assigned as homework to monitor symptoms and skill use. *Behavior chain analyses* are used to review antecedents and consequences of ED behaviors and identify alternative adaptive behaviors. Throughout treatment, the therapist uses a dialectical model that balances accepting the patient for who they are in the moment while pushing for change toward a better life. Therapists use this dialectic to balance validation and warmth with irreverence. *Motivation and commitment strategies* are explicitly used in the pretreatment phase and throughout the course of treatment as individuals' motivation for change waxes and wanes. *Problem-solving strategies* are used in a

2-stage process of first accepting that there is a problem to address and then generating alternative adaptive responses.

Clinical materials/manuals

DBT has been adapted for BN and binge eating in a therapist manual that includes patient handouts.[9] However, the authors recommend first reading the DBT for BPD manuals.[3,10] DBT for binge eating has also been adapted into a guided self-help format.[11]

Empirical Support

Accumulating data provide preliminary support of the efficacy of DBT for BN and BED.[12] To date, there have been no randomized controlled trials (RCTs) of DBT for AN. There have been 2 RCTs in BN, 3 RCTs in BED, and 2 RCTs using transdiagnostic ED samples investigating both a full therapist-led DBT and an abbreviated guided self-help DBT.[12] DBT has been shown to produce better outcomes than wait-list control conditions at the end of treatment,[11,13–16] although there were no differences found at follow-up between DBT and active comparisons.[12]

ACCEPTANCE AND COMMITMENT THERAPY
Theoretic Model

Acceptance and Commitment Therapy (ACT) identifies attempts to escape or avoid distressing internal experiences (eg, thoughts, feelings, or sensations) as a key maintenance factor for psychological disorders.[17] Although many forms of psychotherapy seek to adjust the content of patients' internal experiences as a necessary precursor to behavior change, ACT attempts to shift a patient's relationships with these experiences to facilitate engagement in behaviors more congruent with one's long-term values and goals, even in the presence of aversive internal experiences. As ED behaviors have been conceptualized as maladaptive methods of escaping unpleasant internal states,[18,19] ACT may be particularly well-suited to addressing the observed links between distressing thoughts (eg, "I'm fat") or emotions (eg, negative affect) and ED behaviors.

Structure of the Treatment

Phases/stages

Although ACT explicitly identifies specific psychological processes to be addressed within the course of treatment, the exact order in which these clinical targets are approached is highly flexible and guided by the patient presentation.

Clinical targets/techniques

The primary goal of ACT is to increase psychological flexibility, defined as the ability to continuously adjust one's behaviors in the service of one's chosen values, even when experiencing internal distress. Six therapeutic processes are targeted in pursuit of this goal. *Experiential acceptance* involves embracing one's internal experiences without attempting to change or avoid them. *Defusion* involves creating psychological distance from one's internal momentary experiences. *Present-moment awareness* involves the application of active and flexible attention to the present without judging experiences as good or bad. *Self-as-context*, also referred to as transcendent self-awareness, describes cultivation of a comprehensive sense of self that transcends the idiosyncratic self-images elicited by individual experiences, beliefs, or roles. In other words, individual experiences of the self do not dominate or limit one's overall self-image. *Values clarity* involves identification of one's long-term values (eg, relationships, well-being), which are used as signposts to help guide behaviors toward greater engagement in valued domains. Finally, *committed action* involves setting goals consistent with one's chosen values. Metaphors and experiential exercises are commonly used throughout treatment to help illustrate each of these concepts and assist patients in moving toward greater psychological flexibility.

Clinical materials/manuals

Although ACT has not yet been formally manualized for the treatment of EDs, several helpful texts provide guidance on the delivery of ACT for patients with AN and BN. The 2011 book *Acceptance and Commitment Therapy for Eating Disorders: A Process-Focused Guide to Treating Anorexia and Bulimia* by Sandoz and colleagues[20] provides a thorough review of ACT and EDs as conceptualized by the treatment model, discussion of specific treatment targets and associated exercises, a sample protocol, and various relevant assessments and therapeutic worksheets. A briefer introduction to these concepts can be found in the 2016 compendium *Mindfulness and Acceptance for Treating Eating Disorders and Weight Concerns*, by Haynos and colleagues,[21] which includes an article dedicated to the application of ACT in EDs. Finally, although Heffner and Eifert's[22] 2004 *The Anorexia Workbook: How to Accept Yourself, Heal Your Suffering, and Reclaim Your Life* is written in a self-help format, the patient-friendly text is likely to provide a helpful adjunct to individual or group ACT treatment of individuals with restrictive eating.

Empirical Support

ACT is not currently regarded as an evidenced-based treatment for EDs.[12] Although case series studies suggest that ACT leads to symptom improvement in patients with AN,[23] an RCT found that ACT was not more effective than treatment as usual (TAU) in this population.[24] Similarly, ACT did not outperform TAU among individuals with AN- and BN-spectrum disorders.[25] Finally, a pilot study examining an adaptation of ACT for BED, which incorporates several elements of CBT and DBT, reported post-treatment binge-eating abstinence rates similar to those observed with CBT alone.[26] In sum, the small body of available data suggests that acceptance-based treatments may hold promise as an alternative therapy for EDs. However, the approach has not been demonstrated to be superior to existing treatments, including CBT. Further research is needed to examine the effectiveness of this approach in EDs.

INTEGRATIVE COGNITIVE-AFFECTIVE THERAPY
Theoretic Model

Integrative cognitive-affective therapy (ICAT) offers both a model of ED onset and a separate model for ED maintenance. The model of onset highlights how temperamental variations interact with several factors, such as relationships with others (eg, interpersonal factors) and relationships with the self (self-evaluation, self-regulation) to increase the risk for affective disturbances. It is further posited that such affective disturbances increase the chance of developing ED symptoms. The ICAT maintenance model is momentary in nature and attempts to account for the persistence of ED symptoms over time. Similar to the model of ED onset, interpersonal experiences, situations involving negative self-evaluation, and situations involving hostile and controlling self-regulation strategies are thought to increase momentary emotional dysregulation. Furthermore, it is posited that in the presence of cognitive expectancies, that ED behaviors can reduce the experienced negative affect, ED symptoms are likely to occur. Importantly, it is also predicted that ED symptoms actually do reduce levels of negative affect, but that such reductions are relatively short lived.

Structure of the Treatment

Phases/stages

ICAT has been empirically tested with a 21-session treatment structure spread across 4 phases of treatment. Phase 1, which typically involves 2 to 3 sessions, is focused on enhancing patient education and engagement. Phase 2, which typically includes approximately 5 to 6 sessions, is focused on modifying dietary patterns and managing urges for binge eating and/or purging. Phase 3, which typically involves 10 to 12 sessions, is focused on modifying factors that increase negative emotional arousal, such as problematic relationship patterns, excessive self-evaluation deficits (eg, self-criticism, perfectionism), and maladaptive self-regulation strategies (eg, self-criticism, self-neglect, excessive self-control). Finally, Phase 4, which consists of approximately 2 sessions, is focused on relapse prevention.

Clinical targets/techniques

There are 7 primary targets in ICAT with explicit interventions directed at each. Much of the intervention involves developing skills to engage the target in session, and practicing these skills outside of session. *Emotion identification and awareness skills* involve helping patients to recognize and tolerate different emotional states. *Meal-planning* modules assist patients in reducing meal avoidance and adopting a regular eating pattern. *Binge-eating inhibition skills* are used to help patients engage in adaptive behaviors (eg, self-calming, problem solving) during moments when they are at increased risk of ED behaviors. *Interpersonal skills* are used to assist patients in correcting maladaptive interpersonal patterns (eg, submissiveness, withdrawal) that contribute to ED behaviors. *Self-evaluation skills* support patients in reducing extreme self-evaluation standards in favor of more realistic expectations. *Self-regulation skills* focus on improving patients' self-directed behavior and increasing self-acceptance by reducing patterns of self-criticism, self-neglect, and self-control. *Impulse control and relapse-prevention skills* are incorporated into the final phase of treatment to promote posttreatment management of ED urges and behaviors.

Clinical materials/manuals

The clinical materials used in ICAT include 2 components. The first is a clinician manual, which guides the clinician through the ICAT treatment phases and clinical techniques, using specific instructions and clinical examples.[27] The manual also includes detailed descriptions of the 8 ICAT core skills. In addition to the clinician manual, there is a full complement of patient worksheets included in the published version of the ICAT manual.[27] Patient worksheets are organized according to phase of treatment and provide examples of strategies for promoting target-related change, including an incorporation of affect awareness and meal planning, as well as various self-oriented and other-oriented skills that promote emotion regulation. Mobile versions of the core skills that provide real-time assistance in the natural environment can be downloaded from the Web site at Guilford Publishing (Available at: https://www.guilford.com/books/Integrative-Cognitive-Affective-Therapy-for-Bulimia-Nervosa/Wonderlich-Peterson-Smith/9781462521999/reproducibles).

Empirical Support

Several studies have examined ICAT treatment outcome, as well as moderators of treatment response. In the first study,[28] ICAT was compared with CBT-Enhanced (CBT-E[18]) in the treatment of BN. This study revealed that both ICAT and CBT-E produced clinically meaningful improvements in bulimic psychopathology, associated comorbidity (including depression), and hypothesized maintenance mechanisms including self-discrepancy and emotion regulation, which were maintained at 4-month follow-ups. There were no differences between the 2 treatments on any outcome measure. In addition, 2 studies[29,30] revealed that ICAT was more effective than CBT-E for patients who had high levels of stimulus seeking and affective lability, whereas CBT-E was more effective than ICAT for patients who exhibited low levels of stimulus seeking. Furthermore, evidence suggests that therapeutic alliance was a significant factor in symptom remission for ICAT.[29] The results implied that high levels of therapeutic alliance early in treatment predicated better outcomes, but there was also evidence that change in ED symptoms early in treatment predicted stronger therapeutic alliances later in treatment. This complex relationship highlights the importance of the therapeutic relationship in ICAT.

NEUROCOGNITIVE AND NEUROMODULATION TREATMENTS
Theoretic Model

Neurocognitive and neuromodulation treatments target specific cognitive patterns, regions of the brain, and neural circuits that are thought to be altered among individuals with EDs.[31–33] These interventions have been informed by neurocognitive and neuroimaging data showing specific abnormalities among individuals with EDs in executive functioning, impulse control, reward learning, decision making, central coherence, and cognitive flexibility.[34,35] Neurocognitive treatments, including cognitive remediation treatment (CRT) and attention bias modification, presume that correcting specific types of cognitive processing and attention patterns will result in corresponding clinical improvement. With devices that use electrical current and/or magnetic stimulation, neuromodulation interventions aim to increase or decrease nerve cell activity in neural circuits or brain regions associated with ED psychopathology, including reward and self-regulatory processes.[32,36]

Structure of the Treatment

Phases/stages

Neurocognitive treatments including CRT typically require sequential learning or training sessions in which cognitive exercises or attention bias procedures are practiced repeatedly (eg, weekly for several months). Neuromodulation procedures vary by type. In deep brain stimulation (DBS), electrodes are surgically implanted in specific brain regions to alter neural activity. Noninvasive brain stimulation, including repetitive transcranial magnetic stimulation (rTMS) and transcranial direct current stimulation (tDCS) require recurrent sessions (eg, 5 days each week for 1 to 2 months). For rTMS and tDCS, different brain regions may be targeted depending on symptom presentation. Response to treatment may also impact the duration of treatment.

Clinical targets/techniques

Targets of neurocognitive treatment depend on clinical presentation.[33] For example, CRT can be used to target *cognitive rigidity* in AN. *Attention bias* modification targeting palatable food stimuli can be used to increase inhibitory control among individuals who engage in binge eating. Neuromodulation interventions target specific brain regions and neural circuitry.[32] For example, rTMS and tDCS have been used to target the dorsomedial and the dorsolateral prefrontal cortex because of their importance in *executive functioning* and *inhibitory control*.

Clinical materials/manuals

Neurocognitive treatment requires the completion of cognitive exercises and tasks that can be administered in person or by computer. CRT approaches have been developed to improve cognitive flexibility (eg, being responsive when stimuli change patterns) and central coherence (eg, learning to focus more broadly). Attention bias modification typically uses computer procedures to refocus automatic visual attention from ED-related stimuli (eg, palatable food) to neutral stimuli. DBS requires neurosurgery and ongoing monitoring adjustments based on clinical outcome. rTMS uses electrical current that passes through a magnetic field to increase or suppress brain activity in specific regions. tDCS involves the placement of electrodes on specific regions of the scalp, which deliver electrical current during the completion of a cognitive task or some other type of stimuli to activate specific brain regions or circuits.

Empirical Support

Neurocognitive treatments

Several randomized trials that have been conducted to examine CRT as an adjunctive treatment for AN have observed improvement in cognitive patterns, treatment retention, and clinical presentation.[37,38] Although relatively less research has been conducted using neurocognitive treatment for other types of EDs, preliminary data indicate that attention bias modification may successfully shift visual attention and increase inhibitory control among individuals with binge eating.[33]

Neuromodulation interventions

Several nonrandomized studies of DBS targeting various brain regions (eg, nucleus accumbens) for the treatment of AN have shown promising results.[36] Although preliminary outcome data using rTMS for AN have been associated with clinical improvement, rTMS and tDCS findings for BN are inconsistent.[36]

ADDITIONAL EMERGING PSYCHOLOGICAL TREATMENTS

Third-Wave Behavior Therapy and Mindfulness-Based Interventions

In addition to DBT and ACT, several other third-wave behavior therapies and mindfulness-based interventions are currently being used and adapted for the treatment of EDs. Third-wave and mindfulness-based approaches target the function and awareness of cognitions and emotions, and incorporate mindfulness-based and acceptance-based strategies. These treatments have included compassion-focused therapy, schema therapy, and mindfulness-based interventions. A recent meta-analysis determined that all of these therapies are currently considered possibly efficacious for the treatment of EDs.[12]

Radically open-dialectical behavior therapy (RO-DBT[39]) was developed to target disorders characterized by excessive inhibitory control and has recently been applied to the treatment of AN.[40] Treatment includes individual and skills group sessions that address 5 themes: inhibited and disingenuous emotional expression, overcaution, rigid and rule-governed behavior, aloof and distant interpersonal style, and high social comparison. An initial pilot study of RO-DBT in an inpatient AN sample found improvements in weight gain, and reduction in ED symptoms and related psychopathology.[41]

Treatments Targeting Interpersonal Factors

Couples-based approaches

Family-based treatment is currently the treatment of choice for adolescent AN, suggesting the potential importance of incorporating patients' interpersonal relationships in other treatment approaches. However, until recently, little work had been conducted to address intimate relationships in adult EDs. Although supportive intimate relationships can be central to recovery, many individuals with EDs have difficulty functioning in intimate relationships and cite these relationships as a source of stress rather than support. Although a strict adaptation of family-based treatment strategies would not be developmentally appropriate for most partnered adults (eg, asking patients to relinquish control over food choices to their partners), recent couples-based interventions have adapted cognitive-behavioral couples therapy for application to AN (UCAN[42]) and binge eating (UNITE[43]). Preliminary evidence is promising, supporting the feasibility and acceptability of couples-based approaches for adult EDs.[43,44]

Maudsley anorexia treatment for adults

Maudsley anorexia treatment for adults (MANTRA) is a cognitive-interpersonal treatment for AN, which proposes that factors linked to the underlying obsessional and anxious/avoidant personality traits observed in AN are central to their maintenance. MANTRA uses a motivational interviewing style to address these 4 factors: inflexible thinking style, impairments in the social-emotional domain, beliefs about the positive impact of AN, and unhelpful responses from patients' social support network.[45] MANTRA has been shown to lead to improvements in body mass index, ED symptoms, and clinical impairment in a recent RCT.[46]

Targeting Habit in Eating Disorder Treatment

Regulating emotions and changing habit

The habit model of AN, which conceptualizes restrictive eating as an initially rewarding behavior that becomes an automatic fixed response to specific cues over time,[47] has received initial empirical support.[48] Accordingly, regulating emotions and changing habit (REaCH) is a manualized psychotherapy for EDs that attempts to disrupt relationships between cues and maladaptive behaviors using habit-reversal techniques. The intervention includes 4 phases that address cue-awareness, creation of new routines, suppression of maladaptive habits, and emotion regulation.[49] A recent randomized trial found that, compared with supportive psychotherapy, REaCH was associated with lower global ED symptom severity scores at the end of treatment.[49]

SUMMARY

Although there are currently several evidence-based treatments for EDs, a significant percentage of individuals who receive these interventions drop out of treatment or do not achieve remission at the end of treatment, highlighting the need for novel approaches to fill these gaps. Several promising treatments have recently been adapted or developed to treat EDs based on research exploring emotion regulation, interpersonal factors, and neurocognitive factors that underlie the development and maintenance of ED symptoms. Further research is needed to determine the efficacy and effectiveness of these approaches. Crucial next steps include testing proposed mediators of treatment response to identify clinical targets that confer maximum benefit, and examining moderators of treatment response that may be used to determine optimal patient-specific interventions.

REFERENCES

1. Hilbert A, Hoek HW, Schmidt R. Evidence-based clinical guidelines for eating disorders: international comparison. Curr Opin Psychiatry 2017;30(6):423.
2. National Institute for Health and Care Excellence. Eating disorders: recognition and treatment. NICE Guideline; 2017. Available at: https://www.nice.org.uk/guidance/ng69/resources/eating-disorders-recognition-and-treatment-pdf-1837582159813.
3. Linehan MM. Cognitive behavioral therapy of borderline personality disorder. New York: Guilford Press; 1993.

4. Sloan E, Hall K, Moulding R, et al. Emotion regulation as a transdiagnostic treatment construct across anxiety, depression, substance, eating and borderline personality disorders: a systematic review. Clin Psychol Rev 2017;57:141–63.
5. Lavender JM, Wonderlich SA, Engel SG, et al. Dimensions of emotion dysregulation in anorexia nervosa and bulimia nervosa: a conceptual review of the empirical literature. Clin Psychol Rev 2015;40:111–22.
6. Westwood H, Kerr-Gaffney J, Stahl D, et al. Alexithymia in eating disorders: systematic review and meta-analyses of studies using the Toronto Alexithymia Scale. J Psychosom Res 2017;99:66–81.
7. Oldershaw A, Lavender T, Sallis H, et al. Emotion generation and regulation in anorexia nervosa: a systematic review and meta-analysis of self-report data. Clin Psychol Rev 2015;39:83–95.
8. Wisniewski L, Kelly E. The application of dialectical behavior therapy to the treatment of eating disorders. Cogn Behav Pract 2003;10(2):131–8.
9. Safer DL, Telch CF, Chen EY. Dialectical behavior therapy for binge eating and bulimia. New York: Guilford Press; 2009.
10. Linehan MM. Cognitive-behavioral treatment of borderline personality disorder. New York: Guilford Publications; 2018.
11. Masson PC, von Ranson KM, Wallace LM, et al. A randomized wait-list controlled pilot study of dialectical behaviour therapy guided self-help for binge eating disorder. Behav Res Ther 2013;51(11):723–8.
12. Linardon J, Fairburn CG, Fitzsimmons-Craft EE, et al. The empirical status of the third-wave behaviour therapies for the treatment of eating disorders: a systematic review. Clin Psychol Rev 2017;58:125–40.
13. Courbasson C, Nishikawa Y, Dixon L. Outcome of dialectical behaviour therapy for concurrent eating and substance use disorders. Clin Psychol Psychother 2012;19(5):434–49.
14. Hill DM, Craighead LW, Safer DL. Appetite-focused dialectical behavior therapy for the treatment of binge eating with purging: a preliminary trial. Int J Eat Disord 2011;44(3):249–61.
15. Safer DL, Robinson AH, Jo B. Outcome from a randomized controlled trial of group therapy for binge eating disorder: comparing dialectical behavior therapy adapted for binge eating to an active comparison group therapy. Behav Ther 2010;41(1):106–20.
16. Telch CF, Agras WS, Linehan MM. Dialectical behavior therapy for binge eating disorder. J Consult Clin Psychol 2001;69(6):1061–5.
17. Hayes SC, Strosahl KD, Wilson KG. Acceptance and commitment therapy: the process and practice of mindful change. New York: Guilford Press; 2011.
18. Fairburn CG, Cooper Z, Shafran R, et al. Eating disorders: a transdiagnostic protocol. New York: 2008.
19. Heatherton TF, Baumeister RF. Binge eating as escape from self-awareness. Psychol Bull 1991;110(1):86.
20. Sandoz E, Wilson K, DuFrene T. Acceptance and commitment therapy for eating disorders: a process-focused guide to treating anorexia and bulimia. Oakland (CA): New Harbinger Publications; 2011.
21. Haynos AF, Forman EM, Butryn ML, et al. Mindfulness and acceptance for treating eating disorders and weight concerns: evidence-based interventions. Oakland (CA): New Harbinger Publications; 2016.
22. Heffner M, Eifert GH. The anorexia workbook: how to accept yourself, heal your suffering, and reclaim your life. New York: New Harbinger Publications; 2004.

23. Berman M, Boutelle K, Crow S. A case series investigating acceptance and commitment therapy as a treatment for previously treated, unremitted patients with anorexia nervosa. Eur Eat Disord Rev 2009;17(6):426–34.

24. Parling T, Cernvall M, Ramklint M, et al. A randomised trial of acceptance and commitment therapy for anorexia nervosa after daycare treatment, including five-year follow-up. BMC Psychiatry 2016;16(1):272.

25. Juarascio A, Shaw J, Forman E, et al. Acceptance and commitment therapy as a novel treatment for eating disorders: an initial test of efficacy and mediation. Behav Modif 2013;37(4):459–89.

26. Juarascio AS, Manasse SM, Schumacher L, et al. Developing an acceptance-based behavioral treatment for binge eating disorder: rationale and challenges. Cogn Behav Pract 2017;24(1):1–13.

27. Wonderlich SA, Peterson CB, Smith TL. Integrative cognitive-affective therapy for bulimia nervosa: a treatment manual. New York: Guilford Publications; 2015.

28. Wonderlich SA, Peterson CB, Crosby RD, et al. A randomized controlled comparison of integrative cognitive-affective therapy (ICAT) and enhanced cognitive-behavioral therapy (CBT-E) for bulimia nervosa. Psychol Med 2014; 44(3):543–53.

29. Accurso EC, Wonderlich SA, Crosby RD, et al. Predictors and moderators of treatment outcome in a randomized clinical trial for adults with symptoms of bulimia nervosa. J Consult Clin Psychol 2016;84(2):178–84.

30. Haynos AF, Pearson CM, Utzinger LM, et al. Empirically derived personality sub-typing for predicting clinical symptoms and treatment response in bulimia nervosa. Int J Eat Disord 2017;50(5):506–14.

31. Chen J, Papies EK, Barsalou LW. A core eating network and its modulations underlie diverse eating phenomena. Brain Cogn 2016;110:20–42.

32. Dunlop KA, Woodside B, Downar J. Targeting neural endophenotypes of eating disorders with non-invasive brain stimulation. Front Neurosci 2016;10:30.

33. Eichen DM, Matheson BE, Appleton-Knapp SL, et al. Neurocognitive treatments for eating disorders and obesity. Curr Psychiatry Rep 2017;19(9):62.

34. Lang K, Lopez C, Stahl D, et al. Central coherence in eating disorders: an updated systematic review and meta-analysis. World J Biol Psychiatry 2014;15(8):586–98.

35. Wu M, Hartmann M, Skunde M, et al. Inhibitory control in bulimic-type eating disorders: a systematic review and meta-analysis. PLoS One 2013;8(12):e83412.

36. Dalton B, Campbell IC, Schmidt U. Neuromodulation and neurofeedback treatments in eating disorders and obesity. Curr Opin Psychiatry 2017;30(6):458–73.

37. Dahlgren CL, Rø Ø. A systematic review of cognitive remediation therapy for anorexia nervosa-development, current state and implications for future research and clinical practice. J Eat Disord 2014;2(1):26.

38. Danner UN, Dingemans AE, Steinglass J. Cognitive remediation therapy for eating disorders. Curr Opin Psychiatry 2015;28(6):468–72.

39. Lynch TR. Radically open dialectical behavior therapy: theory and practice for treating disorders of overcontrol. Oakland (CA): New Harbinger Publications; 2018.

40. Hempel R, Vanderbleek E, Lynch TR. Radically open DBT: targeting emotional loneliness in anorexia nervosa. Eat Disord 2018;26(1):92–104.

41. Lynch TR, Gray KL, Hempel RJ, et al. Radically open-dialectical behavior therapy for adult anorexia nervosa: feasibility and outcomes from an inpatient program. BMC Psychiatry 2013;13(1):293.

42. Bulik CM, Baucom DH, Kirby JS, et al. Uniting Couples (in the treatment of) Anorexia Nervosa (UCAN). Int J Eat Disord 2011;44(1):19–28.

43. Runfola CD, Kirby JS, Baucom DH, et al. A pilot open trial of UNITE-BED: a couple-based intervention for binge-eating disorder. Int J Eat Disord 2018; 51(9):1107–12.
44. Baucom DH, Kirby JS, Fischer MS, et al. Findings from a couple-based open trial for adult anorexia nervosa. J Fam Psychol 2017;31(5):584–91.
45. Schmidt UM, Treasure JM. The Maudsley model of anorexia nervosa treatment for adults (MANTRA): development, key features, and preliminary evidence. J Cogn Psychother 2014;28(1):48.
46. Schmidt U, Magill N, Renwick B, et al. The Maudsley outpatient study of treatments for anorexia nervosa and related conditions (MOSAIC): comparison of the Maudsley model of anorexia nervosa treatment for adults (MANTRA) with specialist supportive clinical management (SSCM) in outpatients with broadly defined anorexia nervosa: a randomized controlled trial. J Consult Clin Psychol 2015;83(4):796–807.
47. Walsh BT. The enigmatic persistence of anorexia nervosa. Am J Psychiatry 2013; 170(5):477–84.
48. Foerde K, Steinglass JE, Shohamy D, et al. Neural mechanisms supporting maladaptive food choices in anorexia nervosa. Nat Neurosci 2015;18(11):1571–3.
49. Steinglass JE, Glasofer DR, Walsh E, et al. Targeting habits in anorexia nervosa: a proof-of-concept randomized trial. Psychol Med 2018;48(15):2584–91.

Self-Help Treatment of Eating Disorders

See Heng Yim, BSc[a,*], Ulrike Schmidt, MD, PhD, FRCPsych[a,b]

KEYWORDS

- Self-help • Eating disorders • Review • Bulimia nervosa • Binge eating disorder
- Intervention

KEY POINTS

- Studies of self-help interventions have mainly focused on the treatment of bulimia nervosa (BN), and binge eating disorder (BED), with very few addressing treatment of anorexia nervosa (AN).
- Guided self-help interventions for BN and BED are superior to waiting list or delayed treatment in terms of improving ED psychopathology and abstinence rates.
- Systematic reviews comparing guided self-help (GSH) and other therapies have combined other treatments that are less intensive (pure self-help), more intensive, or equally intensive as GSH. It is hard to draw firm conclusions on the relative efficacy of GSH from these.
- Findings on the impact of guidance on outcome are mixed; however, there is some evidence on the impact of guidance on treatment adherence.
- Future studies are needed to separate out the effects of different modes of self-help (guided/unguided; bibliotherapy/digital), comparison groups (waitlist/type of comparison therapy), as well as the point in the care pathway (prevention, relapse prevention) at which the intervention is delivered.

INTRODUCTION

Self-help programs are structured interventions based on a clear psychological model, which require little or no involvement from a health professional.[1] Currently, most widely evaluated self-help interventions for eating disorders (EDs) are based on disorder-

Disclosure Statement: The First author SHY received salary support from the European Union's Horizon 2020 research and innovation program under grant agreement no 634757. Dr. Schmidt is supported by a Senior Investigator award from the National Institute for Health Research (NIHR) and receives salary support from the NIHR Biomedical Research Centre for Mental Health, South London and Maudsley National Health Service (NHS) Foundation Trust and Institute of Psychiatry, Psychology and Neuroscience, King's College London. The views expressed herein are not those of NIHR or the NHS.
[a] Section of Eating Disorders, King's College London, Institute of Psychiatry, Psychology and Neuroscience, PO Box 59, 16, De Crespigny Park, London SE5 8AF, UK; [b] The Eating Disorders Service, Maudsley Hospital, South London and Maudsley NHS Foundation Trust, London, UK
* Corresponding author.
E-mail address: vanessa.yim@kcl.ac.uk

Table 1
Examples of some empirically evaluated (used in at least 1 RCT) self-help interventions related to EDs

Name	Mode	Example Study
Overcoming binge eating	Book	Dunn et al,[47] 2006
Getting better bite by bite	Book	Schmidt et al,[48] 2007
Working to overcome eating difficulties	Book	Traviss et al,[49] 2011
Overcoming bulimia online	CD-ROM, online	Sánchez-Ortiz et al,[50] 2011
Student bodies+	Online	Beintner et al,[30] 2012
SALUT	Online	Wagner et al,[51] 2013 (SALUT BN); Carrard et al,[42] 2011 (SALUT BED)

specific cognitive behavioral therapy (CBT) (**Table 1**). Only a few feasibility and pilot studies use third-wave CBT principles, such as Acceptance and Commitment Therapy,[2] or Dialectical Behavior Therapy[3] to address the ED, or focus on relevant personality factors (eg, perfectionism) thought to contribute to illness maintenance.[4] Self-help can be administered at various points along the care pathway, ranging from prevention/early intervention, treatment, to relapse prevention/maintenance of recovery.[5] The mode of delivery can be via books or manuals (also known as bibliotherapy), CD-ROMs, videos, or digitally via the Internet and mobile apps. Digital self-help intervention is also referred to as technology-based intervention or as computer-based intervention. This includes Internet-based CBT (iCBT) and computerized CBT. Online delivery is thought to have advantages over other forms due to its scalability[6] and interactivity.[7]

Self-help approaches can be delivered with guidance (guided self-help [GSH]) or without (pure self-help [PSH]). As most self-help interventions are based on CBT, they are also known as CBT-GSH or CBT-PSH. In GSH, the intensity and modality of guidance varies across programs and settings. Guidance can be provided face-to-face, or via email, telephone, or online messaging. As self-help is user-led, the aim of guidance is mainly supportive in nature; it may focus on enhancing motivation and providing clarification, review, and personalization. Some interventions retain the format of face-to-face therapy by having regular weekly guidance sessions, whereas others are briefer and more flexible to allow users to select modules on Web sites or apps. PSH, by contrast, relies entirely on the motivation of the individual user.

Some researchers have argued that self-help interventions are contraindicated in anorexia nervosa (AN) due to the ego-syntonic nature of the disorder and high medical risk.[8,9] However, a small body of evidence suggests that people with AN can benefit from self-help programs enhancing treatment motivation as an adjunct to face-to-face treatment[10,11] or for relapse prevention[12,13] By comparison, self-help is a widely used treatment option for BN and BED where it has a sizable evidence base. In the United Kingdom, guidelines of the National Institute of Care and Excellence recommend self-help interventions as the first step for treatments for "bulimic-type" disorders, including bulimia nervosa (BN), binge eating disorder (BED), and milder forms of binge eating.[14]

The flexible and accessible nature of self-help is believed to reduce barriers to treatment, such as long waiting times, perceived shame and stigma associated with bulimic behaviors, or fear of seeking professional help.[15] From the perspective of the person with the disorder, the user-led nature can empower them by promoting autonomy and independence.[16] From the health care service perspective, self-help interventions can be integrated into a stepped-care approach, whereby people with mild EDs receive low-intensity care and can "step up" for more intensive treatments when needed. This is believed to be less costly than conventional face-to-face therapy as it can be delivered in non-specialist settings.[9]

In the following, the authors present evidence from recent systematic reviews (SRs) and individual randomized controlled trials (RCTs) on the efficacy and effectiveness of different types of self-help interventions. They also summarize what is known about the use of self-help treatments at different stages of the care pathway, their cost-effectiveness, and finally we also look at key factors moderating outcomes. By necessity, the focus will be mainly on interventions focusing on bulimic-type disorders, but where appropriate we will mention other EDs too.

EFFICACY AND EFFECTIVENESS
Findings from Recent Systematic Reviews

Several SRs have summarized the available evidence on self-help interventions for EDs. An early Cochrane SR[17] included bibliotherapy interventions and CD-ROM-based interventions. More recently, there has been an increasing number of reviews on digital self-help.[5,18] **Table 2** summarizes SRs specifically on self-help interventions for EDs published in the last 5 years. In addition, Linardon and colleagues[19] conducted an SR and meta-analysis on the effectiveness of CBT in EDs, which includes CBT self-help. A recent network analysis was published examining the effects of all treatment modalities for BN, again including self-help.[20]

The main outcome measures for intervention efficacy or effectiveness typically include (1) abstinence from ED-related behavioral symptoms, such as bingeing and purging, and (2) reduction in ED psychopathology measured by interview or questionnaires, such as the Eating Disorders Examination Interview[21] or Questionnaire (EDE-Q).[22] Whereas abstinence is widely held to be a "hard" gold standard outcome

Table 2
Systematic reviews on structured stand-alone self-help programs for EDs in the last 5 years

Authors	Studies Evaluated	Type of ED	Type of Self-Help
Aardoom et al,[52] 2013	21 RCTs, controlled studies, uncontrolled studies, qualitative studies until January 2013	All EDs	Internet-based treatment
Beintner et al,[24] 2014	33 RCTs, 1 CT, 16 case series until 2012	BN, BED, EDNOs with binge eating	Manualized GSH & PSH of all modalities
Loucas et al,[18] 2014	20 until July 2014 13 on prevention, 6 on treatment, 1 on relapse prevention	All EDs	Technology-based therapies including CD-ROMs, Internet
Schlegl et al,[5] 2015	22 RCTs, 2 CTs, 16 uncontrolled trials until 2014	All EDs	Technology-based GSH and PSH
Traviss-Turner et al,[23] 2017	30 RCTs until 2016	BN, BED, EDNOs with binge eating	Manualized GSH of all modalities
Pittock et al,[53] 2018	5 RCTs	BN, subthreshold BN or EDNOs-BN (studies that included participants with BED were excluded)	Technology-based CBT

measure, definition of abstinence differs between studies and reviews. For example, whereas Traviss-Turner and colleagues[23] defined abstinence as an absence of behavioral symptoms for 28 days, Beintner and colleagues[24] used the definitions specified in each individual study. Given differences in definitions, unsurprisingly abstinence rates also differ widely across studies. For example, Beintner et al.'s[24] review found between 9% and 64% of the participants to achieve abstinence from bingeing at post-intervention. The effects of the self-help interventions on abstinence are heterogeneous according to several SRs and depend on comparison condition.[19,24]

Self-help interventions versus waiting list

Many studies compare self-help interventions against some kind of waiting list (WL) or delayed treatment condition.

Effects on abstinence Whereas an early Cochrane review[17] did not find any significant difference between WL and intervention group (PSH and GSH combined) on abstinence from bingeing at the end of treatment, the lack of any treatment effect is most likely due to the small number and heterogenous nature of studies available at that time.

In contrast, 3 recent SRs found clear evidence of an effect of self-help on abstinence compared with waiting list.[19,20,23] Traviss-Turner and colleagues[23] found an overall effect in favor of GSH compared with WL on achieving binge abstinence with a small effect size −0.25 (CI [−0.34, −0.15]). A network analysis on treatments of BN[20] found the odds ratio of achieving full remission (defined as being symptom-free for a minimum of 2 weeks) with CBT-GSH compared with WL was 3.81 (credible interval [CrI]: 1.51 to 10.90) and with CBT-PSH was 3.49 (CrI: 1.20–11.21), respectively. There was insufficient evidence to inform a network analysis at longer-term follow-up. The analysis also did not include BED. In addition, for BED, Linardon et al.'s[19] SR found a significant effect of CBT self-help on remission when compared with inactive control at post-treatment. Their SR, however, did not differentiate between PSH and GSH.

Effects on eating disorder psychopathology Findings from different SRs agree that, compared with waitlist controls, both PSH and GSH, whether delivered in book- or technology-based form are superior in improving ED symptoms in BN or BED populations at post-treatment.[17,23]

Self-help versus other treatments

Effects on abstinence The network meta-analysis[20] in BN allowed separate pairwise comparisons between PSH and GSH and between GSH and individual CBT without finding significant differences between these pairs. Another SR by Traviss-Turner and colleagues[23] compared the effect of GSH on abstinence from binge eating with a heterogeneous group of other treatments, including PSH, other GSH treatments or formats (book versus computer-delivered), or face-to-face psychological therapy. Whereas there was a small effect in favor of GSH (relative risk: −0.08 [CI −0.21, 0.04]), these findings are hard to interpret, as some comparison treatments were of lower and others of higher intensity than the GSH interventions.

Effects on eating disorder psychopathology Traviss-Turner and colleagues[23] found a small effect in favor of GSH (relative risk: −0.21 [CI −0.50, 0.07]) when examining the global ED psychopathology. However, for the same reason as above, this finding was difficult to interpret given the heterogeneity in comparison treatments.

In contrast, the SR by Linardon and colleagues[19] did not find significant difference between the effect of CBT self-help on ED psychopathology when compared with other therapies in BED patients. Similar to Traviss-Turner and colleagues,[23] the comparison treatments included a wide range of heterogeneous treatments. There were insufficient studies to examine the effects on BN.

Findings from Key Individual Studies Not Summarized in These Systematic Reviews

A recent large Dutch RCT[25] assigned participants recruited online with self-reported ED symptoms, including those with AN, BN, and BED, to 4 different conditions, with (1) an iCBT program called "featback" consisting of psychoeducation with automated feedback messages, (2) featback with weekly therapist support, (3) featback with 3-times-a-week therapist support, or (4) a WL. Compared with a WL, the featback conditions had small significant effects on reducing bulimic psychopathology, improving mood and reducing perseverative thinking, regardless of the provision and intensity of therapist support. However, those who had some therapist support were more satisfied with their treatment condition than those without.

A recent large-scale multi-center non-inferiority RCT (178 participants) from Germany compared 20 sessions of individual face-to-face CBT with guided iCBT (11 online modules plus 2 × 90-minute sessions with a therapist) for BED.[26] The primary outcome of the study was the difference between groups in objective binge days over the previous 28 days at the end of treatment. In relation to this variable, face-to-face CBT was superior to guided iCBT at end of treatment, and also on abstinence and reduction in ED-related psychopathology at 6-month follow-up. These differences disappeared at 1.5-year follow-up.

Self-Help Studies at Other Stages of the Care Pathway

Several studies have focused on using self-help interventions at different stages of the care pathway, that is, specifically for prevention or early intervention or to prevent relapse after, for example, a period of intensive treatment. These studies exclusively examined iCBT interventions and are summarized below.

Prevention and early intervention

An 8-week, structured iCBT program, StudentBodies, has been widely evaluated in the United States and Germany among female undergraduate students,[27] and those who are at-risk of or have subclinical AN[28] or BED.[29] A meta-analytic review by Beintner and colleagues[30] examined 6 US and 4 German RCTs, and found no clear cultural difference on outcomes. There were mild-to-moderate improvements in ED-related attitudes, on negative body image and desire to be thin scales. The effects were sustained at follow-up. However, a separate SR[18] that included a range of preventative online interventions argued that, across the outcome measures (global ED psychopathology and bulimic symptoms), effect estimates were low for these iCBT programs, including StudentBodies.

The program has been modified and is currently being evaluated in a clinical population in several European countries (Germany, Austria, and United Kingdom).[31]

Relapse prevention

One RCT investigated an Internet relapse prevention program (RP) after inpatient treatment for AN.[27] RP completers gained significantly more weight than treatment-as-usual (TAU), as well as achieving greater reduction in psychopathology (bulimic symptoms on interview, social insecurity, and maturity fears dimensions in EDI-2).

A feasibility trial[13] in the United Kingdom found tentative evidence for the efficacy of a manual-based email-guided self-care program in preventing relapse following inpatient treatment compared with TAU. An RCT by Jacobi and colleagues[32] examined an Internet-based relapse prevention (IN@) for women with BN following inpatient treatment, again compared with TAU. The intervention had a significant effect on vomiting episodes but not on abstinence or binge eating episodes at post-intervention; group differences turned non-significant at follow-up. In a moderator analysis, those who at discharge from inpatient treatment still had bulimic symptoms benefited from the IN@ program, whereas those who were already abstinent did not.

COST-EFFECTIVENESS

Only very few cost-effectiveness studies have focused specifically on self-help treatments for EDs. An SR of such studies identified 13 studies, published until 2017 (Le and colleagues[33]), only 2 of which focused on self-help treatments.[34,35]

One of the studies identified in the SR was part of a Dutch RCT of online self-help with or without therapist guidance, and including a waiting list control, among adults with any type of self-reported ED symptoms.[34] The online intervention seemed to be effective compared with WL; however, there was no clear preference economically regarding the provision of therapist support.

The other study compared book-based CBT-GSH added to TAU with TAU alone in people with BED.[35] This study found CBT-GSH added to TAU was more effective and less costly than TAU alone using both societal and health care perspectives.

Finally, a recent large-scale RCT in women with BED compared the cost-effectiveness of iCBT-GSH with face-to-face individual CBT over a 22-month period.[36] CBT was more effective, but also more costly, compared with iCBT-GSH from a societal perspective. For CBT to be cost-effective, societal willingness to pay had to be high (ie, at least €250 per binge-free day to achieve an 80% probability of being cost-effective).

MODERATORS OF OUTCOME

The heterogeneity of outcomes across studies points to the importance of examining moderating variables. A meta-regression by Beintner and colleagues[24] found a number of such moderators on outcome, including guidance (especially guidance from a specialist), number of guidance sessions, age (which is a proxy of illness duration), body mass index, and severity of ED-related attitudes.

The SR by Traviss-Turner and colleagues[23] found no significant moderating effect of "mode of guidance," "severity of ED," or "amount of contact time," although there was a suggestion that more contact time might be better. They did, however, find that a diagnosis of BED increased the likelihood of abstinence.

The Role of Guidance

In general, the findings relating to the impact of guidance on outcome seem to be mixed. Generalizations and comparisons across studies are difficult to make as many studies do not include information about duration of contact, content of guidance and qualifications of guides/coaches.[5]

Another approach concerns placing guidance as a moderating variable. A meta-regression on self-help interventions for people with "bulimic-type" disorders by Beintner and colleagues[24] indicated that provision of guidance predicted reductions in binge frequency, abstinence from bingeing, and in EDE-Q Eating, Weight, and Shape Concerns. Guidance had the largest impact on ED psychopathology, with GSH yielding larger effect sizes than PSH, assuming similar drop-out and intervention completion rates.

There is stronger evidence on the role of guidance on adherence and satisfaction, which may in turn affect outcome. For example, 1 study reported adherence to self-help at 6% in PSH, and 50% in GSH.[37] Beintner and colleagues[24] found generally lower participation in the PSH condition. Guidance was also associated with higher satisfaction and seen as a helpful element in self-help interventions.[38] Whereas pure self-help can be empowering and enhance autonomy, sufferers may struggle to motivate themselves to persist with this because of perceived lack of support.[39] Treatment motivation can potentially be enhanced through interacting and developing a therapeutic relationship with the guide.[40]

In the light of this evidence, instead of examining the role of guidance per se, perhaps maximizing the helpfulness of guidance should be investigated. Beintner and colleagues[24] proposed the quality of guidance (assessed by the guides' ED expertise) as a moderating variable on outcome and adherence, and found better outcomes when the guide was a specialist. Yet, specialists can be costly. It may be more useful for us to understand the content and quality of good guidance. Qualitative studies showed that reciprocity, trust, and open, strong, and collaborative therapeutic relationships were important for positive treatment outcomes in GSH for BN and BED.[41] Carrard and colleagues[42] interviewed coaches who had high participant retention rates. They reported using a more "therapeutic approach" in their guidance. Interestingly, Sánchez-Ortiz et al.'s[16] content analysis of email guidance in GSH showed that most of the emails had supportive content (95.4%) as opposed to using specific cognitive behavioral techniques.

Treatment Adherence and Drop-Out

Definitions of treatment engagement, adherence, completion, and drop-out vary widely across studies of self-help in EDs. In their review of 4 iCBT studies in ED patients, Fairburn and Murphy[6] found that 16% to 24% of participants did not take up the intervention. In Beintner et al.'s[24] large SR, between 6% and 86% of participants completed the intervention, and between 1% and 88% dropped out. In terms of drop-out at follow-up, another review, specifically on digital self-help, found rates between 4.7% and 84.8%.[5] Across different self-help interventions, bibliotherapy seemed to have the highest participation defined by completion of at least half of the intervention (65%, CI: 54%–75%), followed by CD-ROM (38%, CI: 22%–54%) and Internet-based interventions (37%, CI: 20%–54%).[24] Different reviews found that moderators of drop-out were either inconsistent[38] or could not be determined.[24]

Qualitative studies can give us insights into facilitators of treatment uptake and retention. A small study of online self-help[43] reported reasons for discontinuation of the program to include: lack of motivation, energy, or time; loss of interest; lack of benefits; and technical issues. Some participants are skeptical of self-help for EDs and view this as a "cheap" option with limited or no support.[16,39,40] Other researchers found that a short training presentation increased university students' preference for computerized CBT (CD-ROM) for depression from less than 10% to 30%.[44] It thus seems that managing and communicating expectations helps in optimizing intervention uptake.

SELF-HELP INTERVENTIONS ACROSS CULTURES

Most research on self-help interventions for EDs has been conducted in white girls and women. The evidence base on the acceptability and efficacy in other ethnic groups is limited, although preliminary findings demonstrate the potential of implementing evidence-based self-help programs across cultures. Two small open studies have adapted and tested self-help programs in Mexican Americans[45] and people in Hong Kong.[43]

SUMMARY/IMPLICATIONS

In general, there are multiple barriers to accessing ED care, some of which are patient-related, such as shame, stigma, or secrecy, whereas others are service-related, such as availability or accessibility of specialist treatments. Self-help interventions have the potential for overcoming these barriers, by giving people with EDs timely access to relatively low-cost specialist interventions and empowering them to take charge of their own recovery in the process. Some form of guidance seems to enhance adherence and possibly outcome. However, findings are far from conclusive and many open questions remain. Thus, more research is needed to better understand the place of these interventions in our therapeutic armamentarium. Specifically, we have the following recommendations.

Research Implications

More studies are needed that compare self-help interventions with gold standard face-to-face treatments and include assessments of cost-effectiveness. In addition, further studies of the use of self-help at different stages of the care pathway (eg, from prevention to relapse prevention) would be valuable. We also know very little about the relative merits of book-based versus technology-based interventions. Recent advancements have led to an increase in mobile app-based programs, although most of them are used for self-monitoring purposes.[46] Little is as yet known about the usability and feasibility of delivering mobile-based stand-alone self-help programs. The relative merits of book-based, Web-based, and mobile-based self-help interventions should be further explored.

Very few studies on self-help systematically report adverse events and harms in addition to improvements. Future studies should routinely evaluate these. This will be especially important for self-help interventions with little or no guidance in which clinical risks are less readily monitored.

Clinical Implications

Clinicians who want to offer self-help interventions to their ED patients are well advised to consider how the purpose of and what to expect from a self-help intervention is being communicated to potential users. Other considerations include helping patients set up their use of a self-help intervention in a structured way, to avoid unstructured browsing, and to encourage systematic working through. Careful discussions about these issues, coupled with plans as to what the next steps are, if self-help is not enough to achieve symptom improvement or recovery are needed, to ensure that patients do not feel short-changed.

REFERENCES

1. Lewis G, Anderson L, Araya R, et al. Self-help interventions for mental health problems. Bristol (England): University of Bristol; 2002.

2. Strandskov SW, Ghaderi A, Andersson H, et al. Effects of Tailored and ACT-Influenced Internet-Based CBT for Eating Disorders and the Relation Between Knowledge Acquisition and Outcome: A Randomized Controlled Trial. Behavior Therapy 2017;48(5):624–37.

3. Masson PC, von Ranson KM, Wallace LM, et al. A randomized wait-list controlled pilot study of dialectical behaviour therapy guided self-help for binge eating disorder. Behav Res Ther 2013;51(11):723–8.

4. Steele AL, Wade TD. A randomised trial investigating guided self-help to reduce perfectionism and its impact on bulimia nervosa: a pilot study. Behav Res Ther 2008;46(12):1316–23.

5. Schlegl S, Burger C, Schmidt L, et al. The potential of technology-based psychological interventions for anorexia and bulimia nervosa: a systematic review and recommendations for future research. J Med Internet Res 2015; 17(3):e85.

6. Fairburn CG, Murphy R. Treating eating disorders using the internet. Curr Opin Psychiatry 2015;28(6):461–7.

7. Treasure J, Russell G. The case for early intervention in anorexia nervosa: theoretical exploration of maintaining factors. Br J Psychiatry 2011;199(1):5–7.

8. Tuschen-Caffier B, Herpertz S. Behandlung von Essstörungen: Welche Empfehlungen gibt die S3-Behandlungsleitlinie? Verhaltenstherapie 2012;22(3):191–8.

9. Wilson GT, Zandberg LJ. Cognitive-behavioral guided self-help for eating disorders: effectiveness and scalability. Clin Psychol Rev 2012;32(4):343–57.

10. Brewin N, Wales J, Cashmore R, et al. Evaluation of a motivation and psychoeducational guided self-help intervention for people with eating disorders (MOPED). Eur Eat Disord Rev 2016;24(3):241–6.

11. Fichter M, Cebulla M, Quadflieg N, et al. Guided self-help for binge eating/purging anorexia nervosa before inpatient treatment. Psychother Res 2008;18(5): 594–603.

12. Fichter MM, Quadflieg N, Nisslmüller K, et al. Does internet-based prevention reduce the risk of relapse for anorexia nervosa? Behav Res Ther 2012;50(3): 180–90.

13. Schmidt U, Sharpe H, Bartholdy S, et al. Treatment of anorexia nervosa: a multimethod investigation translating experimental neuroscience into clinical practice. Southampton (United Kingdom): NIHR Journals Library; 2017. Programme Grants for Applied Research, No. 5.16.

14. National Institute for Health and Care Excellence (NICE). Eating disorder: NICE guideline [NG69]. London: NICE; 2017.

15. Becker AE, Hadley Arrindell A, Perloe A, et al. A qualitative study of perceived social barriers to care for eating disorders: perspectives from ethnically diverse health care consumers. Int J Eat Disord 2010;43(7):633–47.

16. Sánchez-Ortiz V, House J, Munro C, et al. "A computer isn't gonna judge you": a qualitative study of users' views of an internet-based cognitive behavioural guided self-care treatment package for bulimia nervosa and related disorders. Eat Weight Disord 2011;16(2):e93–101.

17. Perkins SS, Murphy RR, Schmidt UU, et al. Self-help and guided self-help for eating disorders. Cochrane Database Syst Rev 2006;(3):CD004191.

18. Loucas CE, Fairburn CG, Whittington C, et al. E-therapy in the treatment and prevention of eating disorders: a systematic review and meta-analysis. Behav Res Ther 2014;63:122–31.

19. Linardon J, Wade TD, de la Piedad Garcia X, et al. The efficacy of cognitive-behavioral therapy for eating disorders: a systematic review and meta-analysis. J Consult Clin Psychol 2017;85(11):1080.

20. Slade E, Keeney E, Mavranezouli I, et al. Treatments for bulimia nervosa: a network meta-analysis. Psychol Med 2018;48(16):2629–36.

21. Cooper Z, Fairburn C. The eating disorder examination: a semi-structured interview for the assessment of the specific psychopathology of eating disorders. Int J Eat Disord 1987;6(1):1–8.

22. Fairburn CG, Beglin SJ. Assessment of eating disorders: interview or self-report questionnaire? Int J Eat Disord 1994;16(4):363–70.
23. Traviss-Turner GD, West RM, Hill AJ. Guided self-help for eating disorders: a systematic review and metaregression. Eur Eat Disord Rev 2017;25(3):148–64.
24. Beintner I, Jacobi C, Schmidt UH. Participation and outcome in manualized self-help for bulimia nervosa and binge eating disorder—a systematic review and metaregression analysis. Clin Psychol Rev 2014;34(2):158–76.
25. Aardoom JJ, Dingemans AE, Fokkema M, et al. Moderators of change in an Internet-based intervention for eating disorders with different levels of therapist support: what works for whom? Behav Res Ther 2017;89:66–74.
26. de Zwaan M, Herpertz S, Zipfel S, et al. Effect of internet-based guided self-help vs individual face-to-face treatment on full or Subsyndromal binge eating disorder in overweight or obese patients: the INTERBED randomized clinical trial. JAMA Psychiatry 2017;74(10):987–95.
27. Graff Low K, Charanasomboon S, Lesser J, et al. Effectiveness of a computer-based interactive eating disorders prevention program at long-term follow-up. Eat Disord 2006;14(1):17–30.
28. Taylor CB, Kass AE, Trockel M, et al. Reducing eating disorder onset in a very high risk sample with significant comorbid depression: a randomized controlled trial. J Consult Clin Psychol 2016;84(5):402.
29. Jones M, Luce KH, Osborne MI, et al. Randomized, controlled trial of an internet-facilitated intervention for reducing binge eating and overweight in adolescents. Pediatrics 2008;121(3):453–62.
30. Beintner I, Jacobi C, Taylor CB. Effects of an internet-based prevention programme for eating disorders in the USA and Germany—a meta-analytic review. Eur Eat Disord Rev 2012;20(1):1–8.
31. Vollert B, Beintner I, Musiat P, et al. Using internet-based self-help to bridge waiting time for face-to-face outpatient treatment for Bulimia Nervosa, Binge Eating Disorder and related disorders: study protocol of a randomized controlled trial. Internet Interv 2018;16:26–34.
32. Jacobi C, Beintner I, Fittig E, et al. Web-based aftercare for women with bulimia nervosa following inpatient treatment: randomized controlled efficacy trial. J Med Internet Res 2017;19(9):e321.
33. Le LK-D, Hay P, Mihalopoulos C. A systematic review of cost-effectiveness studies of prevention and treatment for eating disorders. Aust N Z J Psychiatry 2018;52(4):328–38.
34. Aardoom JJ, Dingemans AE, van Ginkel JR, et al. Cost-utility of an internet-based intervention with or without therapist support in comparison with a waiting list for individuals with eating disorder symptoms: a randomized controlled trial. Int J Eat Disord 2016;49(12):1068–76.
35. Lynch FL, Striegel-Moore RH, Dickerson JF, et al. Cost-effectiveness of guided self-help treatment for recurrent binge eating. J Consult Clin Psychol 2010;78(3):322.
36. König HH, Bleibler F, Friederich HC, et al. Economic evaluation of cognitive behavioral therapy and Internet-based guided self-help for binge-eating disorder. Int J Eat Disord 2018;51(2):155–64.
37. Carter JC, Fairburn CG. Cognitive–behavioral self-help for binge eating disorder: a controlled effectiveness study. J Consult Clin Psychol 1998;66(4):616.
38. Aardoom JJ, Dingemans AE, Van Furth EF. E-health interventions for eating disorders: emerging findings, issues, and opportunities. Curr Psychiatry Rep 2016;18(4):42.

39. Pretorius N, Rowlands L, Ringwood S, et al. Young people's perceptions of and reasons for accessing a web-based cognitive behavioural intervention for bulimia nervosa. Eur Eat Disord Rev 2010;18(3):197–206.
40. McClay C-A, Waters L, McHale C, et al. Online cognitive behavioral therapy for bulimic type disorders, delivered in the community by a nonclinician: qualitative study. J Med Internet Res 2013;15(3):e46.
41. Traviss GD, Heywood-Everett S, Hill AJ. Understanding the 'guide'in guided self-help for disordered eating: a qualitative process study. Psychol Psychother 2013; 86(1):86–104.
42. Carrard I, Fernandez-Aranda F, Lam T, et al. Evaluation of a guided internet self-treatment programme for bulimia nervosa in several European countries. Eur Eat Disord Rev 2011;19(2):138–49.
43. Leung SF, Joyce Ma LC, Russell J. An open trial of self-help behaviours of clients with eating disorders in an online programme. J Adv Nurs 2013;69(1):66–76.
44. Mitchell N, Gordon PK. Attitudes towards computerized CBT for depression amongst a student population. Behav Cogn Psychother 2007;35(4):421–30.
45. Shea M, Cachelin FM, Gutierrez G, et al. Mexican American women's perspectives on a culturally adapted cognitive-behavioral therapy guided self-help program for binge eating. Psychol Serv 2016;13(1):31.
46. Anastasiadou D, Folkvord F, Lupianez-Villanueva F. A systematic review of mHealth interventions for the support of eating disorders. Eur Eat Disord Rev 2018;26(5):394–416.
47. Dunn EC, Neighbors C, Larimer ME. Motivational enhancement therapy and self-help treatment for binge eaters. Psychol Addict Behav 2006;20(1):44.
48. Schmidt U, Lee S, Beecham J, et al. A randomized controlled trial of family therapy and cognitive behavior therapy guided self-care for adolescents with bulimia nervosa and related disorders. Am J Psychiatry 2007;164(4):591–8.
49. Traviss GD, Heywood-Everett S, Hill AJ. Guided self-help for disordered eating: a randomised control trial. Behav Res Ther 2011;49(1):25–31.
50. Sánchez-Ortiz V, Munro C, Stahl D. A randomized controlled trial of internet-based cognitive-behavioural therapy for bulimia nervosa or related disorders in a student population. Psychol Med 2011;41:407–17.
51. Wagner G, Penelo E, Wanner C. Internet-delivered cognitive-behavioural therapy vs. conventional guided self-help for bulimia nervosa: long-term evaluation of a randomized controlled trial. Br J Psychiatry 2013;202:135–41.
52. Aardoom JJ, Dingemans AE, Spinhoven P, et al. Treating eating disorders over the internet: a systematic review and future research directions. Int J Eat Disord 2013;46(6):539–52.
53. Pittock A, Hodges L, Lawrie SM. The effectiveness of internet-delivered cognitive behavioural therapy for those with bulimic symptoms: a systematic review. BMC Res Notes 2018;11(1):748.

Clinician-Delivered Teletherapy for Eating Disorders

Laura Elizabeth Sproch, PhD, Kimberly Peddicord Anderson, PhD*

KEYWORDS

- Teletherapy • Telepsychotherapy • Telepsychology • Eating disorder
- Telemedicine • Videoconferencing • Telemental health • Psychotherapy

KEY POINTS

- Videoconferencing (VC) psychotherapy is a means of improving access to evidence-based ED care for those in need.
- Research suggests that the application of evidence-based protocols using teletherapy formats leads to significant improvement of ED symptoms and associated problems; however, additional research is necessary.
- Specific administrative considerations, including legal issues, patient environment, and technology access, exist for ED teletherapy and require close examination before implementing such treatment.
- Therapeutic alliance, satisfaction, and safety issues are comparable between ED in-person and VC therapy, with notable exceptions. Recognition of the clinical benefits specific to teletherapy, and counterindications, is essential.
- The importance of therapist training before the application of VC psychotherapy cannot be overstated.

INTRODUCTION

The mental health field has progressed and evolved to accommodate for its clinical population, the ever-changing culture, and advancing scientific knowledge. The turn to evermore specialist care is one example of such adaptation. Time has shown that distinct clinical issues often require distinct evidence-based treatment and specialized training. The treatment of eating disorders (EDs) is no exception. In fact, evidence-based ED treatment particularly highlights the importance of specialist care requiring mandatory education, training, supervision, and experience.[1–3] One

Disclosures: The authors have no disclosures of relationships with a commercial company that has a direct financial interest in subject manner or materials discussed in this article or with a company making a competing product.
Department of Psychology, The Center for Eating Disorders at Sheppard Pratt, 6535 North Charles Street, Suite 300, Baltimore, MD 21204, USA
* Corresponding author.
E-mail address: KAnderson@sheppardpratt.org

Psychiatr Clin N Am 42 (2019) 243–252
https://doi.org/10.1016/j.psc.2019.01.008
0193-953X/19/© 2019 Elsevier Inc. All rights reserved.

obvious barrier to implementing ED-specialized psychotherapy is that in large pockets of North America, access to well-trained ED therapists can seem impossible. This produces two critical issues: EDs treated by providers not well-trained in evidence-based treatment, and lack of initiation of care by those in need because services are not easily identified and accessed. Research shows that for the most part, EDs go untreated. Individuals instead receive treatment of other mental health conditions or obesity and from providers (eg, primary care physicians) without requisite training in ED treatment protocols.[4–6] Sparked by the technology boom and its never-ending quest for staying current, the mental health field has recognized this accessibility issue and started using technology to disseminate treatment. Behavioral health treatment delivered through the Internet allows clinicians to offer face-to-face treatment with patients remotely located. This article informs clinicians of the utility, feasibility, and special considerations of using teletherapy for ED-specialized care.

First, we must focus the terminology used in this article because the term "teletherapy" is broad. In previous work, teletherapy has included videoconferencing (VC), telephone services, email therapy, text therapy, smartphone applications, virtual reality, and guided and unguided self-help (through software and online programs). Numerous recent reviews have been conducted that outline a combination of a variety of these teletherapy services for EDs.[7–11] This article focuses exclusively on therapist-delivered psychotherapy for clinical EDs via VC and exclude alternate forms listed previously. We have selected this mode in particular because we believe it to be the most duplicative of in-person protocols for clinical EDs with an established strong evidence base. Self-help treatment is an exception to this statement because the efficacy of this treatment of particular ED presentations is clear and is well reviewed in another article of this issue (See Heng Yim and Ulrike Schmidt's article, "Self-help Treatment of Eating Disorders," in this issue).

EVIDENCE FOR TELETHERAPY
General Psychotherapy

Within the past 15 years, substantial implementation and evaluation of teletherapy in general clinical populations has occurred. In their review, Hilty and colleagues[12] concluded that for the most part, teletherapy is comparable with in-person treatment of adult depression and anxiety. According to Backhaus and colleagues,[13] therapist-delivered VC psychotherapy in particular tends to be feasible, can reduce burden, is satisfactory for patients, and leads to clinical symptom reduction in nonrandomized controlled clinical trials. Randomized controlled studies suggest that cognitive-behavioral therapy (CBT) for childhood depression,[14] psychiatric treatment including brief supportive counseling for adult depression,[15] family counseling for epilepsy,[16] anger management CBT group therapy for adults,[17] and CBT group therapy for post-traumatic stress disorder[18] produces similar clinical symptom change between in-person and VC psychotherapy.

Specialized Eating Disorder Treatment

One randomized controlled trial of therapist-delivered teletherapy for ED-specialized care has been conducted. Mitchell and colleagues[19] randomly assigned 128 adults diagnosed with either bulimia nervosa or ED not otherwise specified (with binge eating or purging at least once per week) to VC or in-person CBT. In the in-person condition, CBT therapists traveled to the participant's local community to provide therapy, whereas in the VC condition, participants received services via computer at a local health care facility. Results showed no statistically significant between-group differences in attrition; abstinence rates of objective binge eating, purging, and combined binge eating/purging; ED restraint and weight concern; self-esteem; and quality of life. Compared with the VC condition, participants in the in-person condition had significantly less frequent binge eating and purging episodes. That is, at baseline, VC participants endorsed 19.1 objective binge eating episodes over the course of 28 days, which decreased to 6.2 at end of treatment. In the in-person condition, episodes decreased from 21.9 to 3.7 during the same timeframe. For purging episodes, VC participants decreased from 36.8 to 11.1 episodes in a 28-day period, whereas those in the in-person condition decreased from 35.6 to 5.6. Of note, at 12-month follow-up, binge eating frequency was found to be no longer significant between conditions; however, purging frequency differences were significant in that VC participants' number of episodes was 19.4 compared with the in-person condition, which was 8.2. Response to treatment measured by reduction in bingeing and purging frequency occurred more rapidly in the in-person condition compared with the VC condition, which had a more gradual response. Results indicated that there were significant group differences (ie, participants receiving in-person treatment scoring at lower levels) at 12-month follow-up on shape concerns, at 3-month follow-up on eating concerns, and at treatment end on depression symptoms. Despite these findings, the authors summarize that the treatments were "roughly equivalent" because of minimally significant differences. In follow-up studies, results indicated that, compared with the in-person condition, the VC condition was associated with the benefit of lower costs.[20] Additionally, predictors of treatment response differences were found between conditions, suggesting earlier symptom change in the VC condition, compared with the in-person condition.[21] Also, although therapists' ratings of therapeutic alliance were lower in earlier stages of treatment, patients' reports of therapeutic alliance were similar in the VC and in-person conditions.[22]

A few studies have evaluated VC psychotherapy for EDs without control conditions. Family-based treatment of adolescents was found to be feasible and acceptable and led to increased weight, decreased eating pathology, and decreased depressive symptoms from baseline to end of treatment and to 6-month follow-up.[23] VC application of CBT for EDs has been shown to be satisfying for patients and has led to decreased ED symptoms, decreased depression, and improved nutritional knowledge.[24–26]

TELETHERAPY CONSIDERATIONS FOR EATING DISORDER CARE
Administrative Considerations

Teletherapy laws, regulations, consent, and licensure
In the United States, current federal law dictates Medicare coverage of teletherapy at the same rate as in-person treatment.[27] Certain restrictions apply, such as the requirement that patients are seen at an originating site (eg, local clinic setting, community health center, and hospital) and that a patient can only receive telemental health care if located within a health professional shortage area or outside a metropolitan statistical area. State law controls regulations for Medicaid and private insurers. As of 2018, telehealth parity laws have been adopted in 36 states requiring managed care companies to cover teletherapy at the same rate as in-person treatment. Specific coverage and training/documentation requirements vary depending on insurance provider and state regulations. If teletherapy is not a covered benefit within an insurance plan but access to ED-specialized care is not readily available, at times special approvals are made to cover such services. Because of the special considerations required for teletherapy services, a separate consent form is recommended. Close

review of the consent form by a provider with the patient is likely necessary to ensure agreement and understanding. Many of the topics reviewed in this article could be specifically included in a consent form (**Box 1**).

Regarding licensure, consultation with a therapist's professional board may help to ascertain where a clinician or patient needs to be located and licensed in order for services to be rendered. For example, in Maryland, a psychologist needs to be licensed in the state where a patient is physically located during a session to provide covered services. The Association of State and Provincial Psychology Boards' Psychology Interjurisdictional Compact (PSYPACT) is an interstate agreement created to facilitate treatment across state lines.[28] This agreement allows psychologists in PSYPACT-enacted states to treat patients located in states in which they are not licensed.

Teletherapist training

Training on specific considerations for the implementation of teletherapy is paramount. There are multiple telemedicine professional organizations on an international and national level that offer expert resources. In particular, the American Telemedicine Association is the leading American telehealth association that, among other contributions, offers a variety of educational opportunities, including courses, webinars, and trainings on telemedicine topics for providers. The American Telemedicine Association's *Practice Guidelines for Videoconferencing-Based Telemental Health*[29] and the American Psychological Association's *Guidelines for the Practice of Telepsychology*[30] provide practical considerations for teletherapy implementation. Additionally, state- and

---

Box 1
Consent form topics recommended for teletherapy for EDs

Intention and purpose of teletherapy

Explanation of differences between teletherapy and in-person care

Eligibility criteria for teletherapy services

Specific minimum technology requirements

Limits of confidentiality in electronic communication

Technology backup plan

Establishment of a private therapy space

Privacy issues (eg, use of mobile devices for sessions or alerting provider if someone else is present)

Limits of session location based on state policy

Communication plan related to location changes

Safety management and identification of an emergency management plan

Identification of a support person

Medical management plan

Situations in which a teletherapy session would be discontinued

Appropriateness of session recordings

Risks and benefits

Alternatives to teletherapy

Circumstances in which teletherapy would not be warranted and plan for in-person services

regional-level telemedicine organizations and resource centers support providers with particular needs related to their geographic area. ED-specific organizations, such as the Academy for Eating Disorders, can offer additional support on the topic of teletherapy within the area of EDs.

Patient environment

There are two versions of teletherapy that affect the environment in which a patient receives care. In some forms of VC teletherapy, the patient travels to an originating site where the individual uses a VC-connected office space to receive therapy services by a clinician remotely located. There are many benefits of this type of arrangement. Most importantly, is the availability of the originating site's staff members in case of an emergency, and the capability to manage paperwork and billing needs and to coordinate with a general practitioner on medical issues. The alternative setup is to have a patient use their own technology (eg, personal computer) to receive services in their personal environment. Obvious benefits of this variation include convenience for the patient and the clinician in that no additional relationship needs to be established with an office distantly located. In this version of teletherapy, special consideration may need to be given to the patient's chosen physical environment during a session. Private and confidential locations are required (eg, private office spaces or homes) where a patient believes that they can speak freely without the risk of someone overhearing therapy material. It should be made clear that patients should not have anyone else present in the session, unless discussed as a part of a treatment plan. The confidentiality of the space may need to be reevaluated regularly and problem solving conducted when needed. Considerations related to what type of technology (eg, personal computer, laptop, tablet, or smartphone) is important because portability of such devices may affect location and confidentiality.

Technology and technological issues

To provide adequate teletherapy services, specific recommendations for the provider and patient include: professional grade and reliable high-quality equipment (ie, cameras, microphones, monitors, computers, and speakers), up-to-date antivirus software, personal firewall, adequate bandwidth, and high-speed Internet.[29,30] It is recommended that providers and patients test their technology before an initial session and equipment limitations (eg, poor camera resolution or inadequate lighting) be addressed immediately because any disruption in technology could distract from treatment or lead to premature termination of sessions. In the rare event of a complete technical failure, a backup plan agreed on at the start of treatment may be helpful for the patient and provider. Such a plan could include the temporary transition to voice-only communication.

Close consideration of a well-suited VC platform is necessary. In the United States, a VC platform needs to be compliant with the Health Insurance Portability and Accountability Act (HIPAA) and therefore is required to be confidential and secure, which includes private connections or encryption. Many popular VC platforms that are not designed specifically for health care services are not HIPAA compliant. Some insurers have an approved list of VC platforms. Typically, platforms have a monthly or annual rate depending on the number of clients or providers using the service and/or access to particular features. It is advised to consider the method in which a teletherapist will coordinate sharing documents (eg, administrative forms, consent forms, or therapy worksheets) with the patient, such as using a HIPAA-compliant file share program through the VC platform. Computer scanners or scanner apps may be required. As in face-to-face therapy, clinicians should have guidelines regarding use of email or text messages in the provision of care.

Clinical Considerations

Therapeutic alliance and patient and therapist satisfaction

Teletherapy seems to be well-accepted and patients are satisfied with this delivery method overall[13,22]; however, more research in this area is needed.[31] Clinicians should remain alert to potential influences of VC treatment on the therapeutic alliance. For example, VC's lack of an in-office structure, potential reduced ability to hear vocal tone, inability to astutely read body language, and risk of technical problems have been identified as possible areas of concern. As a result, some patients may be less likely to establish a therapeutic alliance remotely than others. Furthermore, there may be certain aspects of the therapeutic alliance (eg, trust) that are more difficult to develop with remote therapy delivery, although this is an area needing more investigation.[18] In other areas of telehealth, patients seem to prefer a combination of in-person therapy and online sessions versus online sessions alone.[32] For some, blending treatment in this way might allow for the full development of the therapeutic alliance while receiving the benefits of teletherapy.

Given the expectation that teletherapy will continue to expand within the field, therapists' apprehension with providing remote treatment coupled with potential difficulty developing early therapeutic alliance[22] needs to be addressed. The expressed concerns may be the result of inexperience with VC, discomfort with technology, or a general doubt about the VC delivery method. Additional therapist training may be needed. It has been found that comfort and satisfaction with teletherapy by providers increases throughout the course of treatment.[22] Nevertheless, if the therapeutic alliance between the therapist and patient does not become well established, treatment may suffer because it could affect patient openness, self-disclosure, and outcome. If it is perceived by the patient or therapist that the alliance is suffering because of the remote intervention, a transition to in-person therapy is recommended.

Safety

With teletherapy, the management of high-risk patients may pose a unique challenge to the clinician; however, when prepared with emergency protocols, addressing safety through VC has been shown to be safe and effective.[33,34] Therapists treating EDs need to adhere to general teletherapy guidelines[29] and may require additional, more specific, planning for safety with this population. ED teletherapists are necessarily assessing eating, weight, mood, suicidality, self-harm, substance use, and other dangerous behaviors on a regular basis to follow best practices for safe ED treatment.[1–3] Although a high reliability between in-person and VC assessments, across diagnoses, has been demonstrated,[35] there may be some information that is more difficult to obtain (eg, smell of alcohol or subtle scratches from self-harm). As a result, it is recommended that therapists have a low threshold when asking about such behaviors and that assessments, including standardized measures, continue routinely throughout treatment.[36] Obtaining weights for patients with EDs is often a mandatory component of assessment, treatment, and safety monitoring and requires that a teletherapist develops a unique plan to obtain such information. For example, a therapist may ask patients to weigh themselves while observing the process, ask family members to obtain weights and report them through the platform, or require patients to be weighed at a primary care physician's office or the originating site clinic. For the assessment of suicidality or self-harm in teletherapy, it is recommended that a specific emergency plan be written down and discussed fully before initiating therapy.[36] This plan would include the names and contact numbers of a local support person, medical providers, and available community emergency systems, and the terms under which these supports would be contacted. Some have recommended that the teletherapist have a second clinician available to provide assistance with coordination of the care (eg, talking to police or calling 9-1-1) during a crisis situation.[37] Emergency preparedness also includes a familiarity with federal, state, and local laws regarding commitment requirements and duty to warn/protect.

Given the nutritional and medical complications that are associated with EDs, coordination of care with primary medical providers is also an important aspect of safety planning. There will likely be numerous occasions for coordination with primary care physicians, especially for patients with more severe EDs. For instance, it is not uncommon for ED therapists to monitor vital signs at the time of a therapy session, using nursing assistance, when a concern arises; however, this is not possible in a VC session. Although immediate assessment of vitals is ideal in such circumstances, teletherapists instead may need to contact the patient's primary medical provider and ask the patient to be seen as soon as possible. If an agreed on pretreatment plan related to medical monitoring is in place, this could prevent patient delay in following through with such recommendations.

Unique clinical benefits

The benefits of teletherapy are clear. It is cost effective, convenient, and most importantly, provides the opportunity for empirically supported treatment to those without access.[12] Beyond this, key clinical benefits specific to ED treatment have been detected. For example, family meals, environmental modifications, and various behavioral exposures can be conducted in vivo, with therapist support. With teletherapy, as a therapist observes and facilitates, a patient may discard diet products, modify mirrors, prepare and complete an exposure food item, remove exercise equipment, or post grocery lists/menus in a kitchen, all interventions typically discussed as a part of CBT for EDs. In a family meal intervention, meal preparation may be substantially easier, because there may be greater flexibility with menu options, more family members may be available, and families can practice in their natural environment. Finally, clinicians have observed that teletherapy seems to be especially suited for patients with less severe illness. A stepped-care approach for EDs involving teletherapy has been discussed[38] and seems to occur organically in some situations. For instance, for college-aged patients, teletherapy is much more acceptable to the busy student with mild symptoms who is not convinced about the need for treatment. Similarly, for the student returning to college following significant improvement with treatment, teletherapy may allow care to continue uninterrupted.

Clinical indicators that teletherapy may not be appropriate

Despite the growing literature suggesting that teletherapy is an effective and safe way to deliver mental health treatment,[12,19] there may be situations where it is not appropriate. Considerations include patient and therapist comfort level with the out of office environment (discussed previously), a history of repeated in-therapy crisis or problematic behaviors, severe and/or worsening symptoms, follow through with medical care requirements, therapeutic alliance issues, and the level of engagement required for effective therapy.[30,36]

SUMMARY AND FUTURE DIRECTIONS

For clinicians treating EDs, teletherapy is a new field. Because the current body of evidence is limited in scope and methodology,[39] it is recommended that teletherapy not be used as a substitute for traditional in-person therapy when this format is available. It is, however, strongly recommended in situations where there is a compelling reason for this form of treatment, such as a patient's inability to access evidence-based ED treatments within a manageable traveling distance. Many individuals across North America are in such circumstances and it is the hope that there will be a growing application of teletherapy to accommodate those in need. Specific administrative and clinical applications, discussed in this article, are paramount when considering this mode of treatment. There is much future research to be done, including evaluating evidence-based ED treatments, across diagnoses, in randomized controlled trials comparing in-person therapy, VC psychotherapy, and waitlist controls with follow-up data collection. Additional research is required to reevaluate compliance, therapeutic alliance, and comfort with VC psychotherapy as the culture becomes increasingly habituated to technology use. Also, research examining differing age groups, ED group treatment formats, and whether specific interventions may be more efficacious in a teletherapy format (eg, behavioral interventions may be more effective because of in vivo exposure benefits) is indicated.

REFERENCES

1. National Institute for Health and Care Excellence (NICE). Eating disorders: recognition and treatment. NICE guideline 69. 2017. Available at: http://nice.org.uk/guidance/ng69. Accessed October 29, 2018.
2. Yager J, Devlin MJ, Halmi KA, et al. Guideline watch (August 2012): practice guideline for the treatment of patients with eating disorders. 3rd edition. Arlington (VA): American Psychiatric Association; 2012. Available at: https://psychiatryonline.org/pb/assets/raw/sitewide/practice_guidelines/guidelines/eatingdisorders-watch.pdf. Accessed October 29, 2018.
3. Yager J, Devlin MJ, Halmi KA, et al. Practice guideline for the treatment of patients with eating disorders. 3rd edition. Arlington (VA): American Psychiatric Association; 2006. Available at: http://psychiatryonline.org/pb/assets/raw/sitewide/practice_guidelines/guidelines/eatingdisorders.pdf. Accessed October 29, 2018.
4. Cachelin FM, Rebeck R, Veisel C, et al. Barriers to treatment for eating disorders among ethnically diverse women. Int J Eat Disord 2001;30(3):269–78.
5. Cachelin FM, Striegel-Moore RH. Help seeking and barriers to treatment in a community sample of Mexican American and European American women with eating disorders. Int J Eat Disord 2006;39(2):154–61.
6. Mond JM, Hay PJ, Rodgers B, et al. Health service utilization for eating disorders: findings from a community-based study. Int J Eat Disord 2007;40(5): 399–408.
7. Agras WS, Fitzsimmons-Craft EE, Wilfley DE. Evolution of cognitive-behavioral therapy for eating disorders. Behav Res Ther 2017;88:26–36.
8. Anastasiadou D, Folkvord F, Lupiañez-Villanueva F. A systematic review of mHealth interventions for the support of eating disorders. Eur Eat Disord Rev 2018;26(5):294–416.
9. Fairburn CG, Murphy R. Treating eating disorders using the Internet. Curr Opin Psychiatry 2015;28(6):461–7.
10. Fairburn CG, Rothwell ER. Apps and eating disorders: a systematic clinical appraisal. Int J Eat Disord 2015;48(7):1038–46.
11. Schlegl S, Bürger C, Schmidt L, et al. The potential of technology-based psychological interventions for anorexia and bulimia nervosa: a systematic review and recommendations for future research. J Med Internet Res 2015;17(3):e85.

12. Hilty D, Yellowlees PM, Parrish MB, et al. Telepsychiatry: effective, evidence-based, and at a tipping point in health care delivery? Psychiatr Clin North Am 2015;38(3):559–92.

13. Backhaus A, Agha Z, Maglione ML, et al. Videoconferencing psychotherapy: a systematic review. Psychol Serv 2012;9(2):111–3.

14. Nelson EL, Barnard M, Cain S. Treating childhood depression over videoconferencing. Telemed J E Health 2003;9(1):49–55.

15. Ruskin PE, Silver-Aylaian M, Kling MA, et al. Treatment outcomes in depression: comparison of remote treatment through telepsychiatry to in-person treatment. Am J Psychiatry 2004;161(8):1471–6.

16. Glueckauf RL, Fritz SP, Ecklund-Johnson EP, et al. Videoconferencing-based family counseling for rural teenagers with epilepsy: phase one findings. Rehabil Psychol 2002;47(1):49–72.

17. Morland LA, Greene CJ, Rosen CS, et al. Telemedicine for anger management therapy in a rural population of combat veterans with posttraumatic stress disorder: a randomized noninferiority trial. J Clin Psychiatry 2010;71(7):855–63.

18. Frueh BC, Monnier J, Yim E, et al. A randomized trial of telepsychiatry for post-traumatic stress disorder. J Telemed Telecare 2007;13(3):142–7.

19. Mitchell JE, Crosby RD, Wonderlich SA, et al. A randomized trial comparing the efficacy of cognitive–behavioral therapy for bulimia nervosa delivered via telemedicine versus face-to-face. Behav Res Ther 2008;46(5):581–92.

20. Crow SJ, Mitchell JE, Crosby RD, et al. The cost effectiveness of cognitive behavioral therapy for bulimia nervosa delivered via telemedicine versus face-to-face. Behav Res Ther 2009;47(6):451–3.

21. Marrone S, Mitchell JE, Crosby R, et al. Predictors of response to cognitive behavioral treatment for bulimia nervosa delivered via telemedicine versus face-to-face. Int J Eat Disord 2009;42(3):222–7.

22. Ertelt TW, Crosby RD, Marino JM, et al. Therapeutic factors affecting the cognitive behavioral treatment of bulimia nervosa via telemedicine versus face-to-face delivery. Int J Eat Disord 2011;44(8):687–91.

23. Anderson KE, Byrne CE, Crosby RD, et al. Utilizing telehealth to deliver family-based treatment for adolescent anorexia nervosa. Int J Eat Disord 2017;50(10): 1235–8.

24. Bakke B, Mitchell J, Wonderlich S, et al. Administering cognitive-behavioral therapy for bulimia nervosa via telemedicine in rural settings. Int J Eat Disord 2001; 30(4):454–7.

25. Simpson S, Bell L, Britton P, et al. Does video therapy work? A single case series of bulimic disorders. Eur Eat Disord Rev 2006;14(4):226–41.

26. Simpson S, Knox J, Mitchell D, et al. A multidisciplinary approach to the treatment of eating disorders via videoconferencing in north-east Scotland. J Telemed Telecare 2003;9(Suppl 1):S37–8.

27. Centers for Medicare and Medicaid Services. Telehealth services, Medicare learning network. Baltimore (MD): Dept of Health and Human Services; 2018. Available at: https://www.cms.gov/Outreach-and-Education/Medicare-Learning-Network MLN/MLNProducts/downloads/TelehealthSrvcsfctsht.pdf. Accessed October 29, 2018.

28. Webb C, Orwig J. Expanding our reach: telehealth and licensure implications for psychologists. J Clin Psychol Med Settings 2015;22(4):243–50.

29. Yellowlees P, Shore JH, Roberts L. American Telemedicine Association: practice guidelines for videoconferencing-based telemental health. Telemed J E Health 2010;16(10):1074–89.

30. Joint Task Force for the Development of Telepsychology Guidelines for Psychologists. Guidelines for the practice of telepsychology. Am Psychol 2013;68(9): 791–800.
31. Whitten PS, Mair F. Telemedicine and patient satisfaction: current status and future directions. Telemed J E Health 2000;6(4):417–23.
32. McClay CA, Waters L, McHale C, et al. Online cognitive behavioral therapy for bulimic type disorders, delivered in the community by a nonclinician: qualitative study. J Med Internet Res 2013;15(3):e46.
33. Luxton DD, Sirotin AP, Mishkin MC. Safety of telemental healthcare delivered to clinically unsupervised settings: a systematic review. Telemed J E Health 2010; 16(6):705–11.
34. Luxton DD, June JD, Kinn JT. Technology-based suicide prevention: current applications and future directions. Telemed J E Health 2011;17(1):50–4.
35. Shore J. Telepsychiatry: videoconferencing in the delivery of psychiatric care. Am J Psychiatry 2013;170(3):256–62.
36. Luxton DD, O'Brien K, McCann RA, et al. Home-based telemental healthcare safety planning: what you need to know. Telemed J E Health 2012;18(8):629–33.
37. Gros DF, Yoder M, Tuerk PW, et al. Exposure therapy for PTSD delivered to veterans via telehealth: predictors of treatment completion and outcome and comparison to treatment delivered in person. Behav Ther 2011;42(2):276–83.
38. Myers TC, Swan-Kremeier L, Wonderlich S, et al. The use of alternative delivery systems and new technologies in the treatment of patients with eating disorders. Int J Eat Disord 2004;36(2):123–43.
39. Aardoom JJ, Dingemans AE, Van Furth EF. E-health interventions for eating disorders: emerging findings, issues, and opportunities. Curr Psychiatry Rep 2016; 18(42):2–8.

Pharmacologic Treatment of Eating Disorders

Scott J. Crow, MD[a,b,*]

KEYWORDS

- Eating disorders • Anorexia nervosa • Bulimia nervosa • Binge eating disorder
- Medication • Fluoxetine

KEY POINTS

- Medication plays a very limited role in the treatment of anorexia nervosa.
- Numerous antidepressants can be used to treat bulimia nervosa.
- High-dose fluoxetine (ie, 60 mg/d) is the standard of care medication approach for BN.
- Numerous medications can treat binge eating disorder but tend to bring little change in weight.

INTRODUCTION

Psychopharmacologic agents can play an important role in the treatment of eating disorders. However, the role of medication treatment of eating disorders differs from that seen in other areas of psychiatric treatment. Medications are a key treatment approach for many psychiatric illnesses (for example, schizophrenia or bipolar illness). However, they do not play this same role in eating disorders. Generally, medications follow in importance behind nutritional approaches and psychotherapy. Nonetheless, there is a longstanding, fairly substantial literature on the impact of medications for various eating disorder symptoms. Furthermore, there is evidence, at least for bulimia nervosa (BN), that including medication early in the treatment algorithm in a stepped care approach may be cost-effective.[1]

The role of medication varies considerably by eating disorder diagnosis. Carefully conducted studies examining the impact of medications on anorexia nervosa (AN) and BN date back to the 1980s, and, in more recent years, the use of medications for binge eating disorder (BED) has been an active area of inquiry. In the case of BN and BED, a U.S. Food and Drug Administration (FDA)-approved medication exists for each, with many other studies showing benefit for a wide variety of other medications. The treatment of AN differs; the degree of benefit shown in most studies to date has been quite limited.

Disclosure Statement: None.
[a] Department of Psychiatry, University of Minnesota, F282/2A West, 2450 Riverside Avenue, Minneapolis, MN 55434, USA; [b] The Emily Program, St Paul, MN 55108, USA
* F282/2A West, 2450 Riverside Avenue, Minneapolis, MN 55454.
E-mail address: crowx002@umn.edu

Psychiatr Clin N Am 42 (2019) 253–262
https://doi.org/10.1016/j.psc.2019.01.007
0193-953X/19/© 2019 Elsevier Inc. All rights reserved.

psych.theclinics.com

This article reviews the existing literature on medication treatment of AN, BN, and BED. Options, goals for treatment, and general strategy are examined. The potential impact of medications on avoidant/restrictive food intake disorder (ARFID) and other specified eating disorders (OSFED) are also briefly discussed.

GENERAL CONSIDERATIONS AND STRATEGY
When to Consider Medication Treatment

There are several instances in which medication treatment should be considered for the management of people who have eating disorders. First, medications should be considered when other treatments (particularly psychotherapy) have not worked well enough.

Second, medications can be uniquely valuable when geography limits access to specialized treatment. In many regions, travel of at least several hours is needed to reach a clinician who can provide specialized eating disorder-focused psychotherapy. By contrast, pharmacies are nearly everywhere, and medications are readily available via mail-order pharmacy. Moreover, psychiatrists and primary care providers providing medication treatment are far more widely distributed than are eating disorder specialist psychotherapists. These factors render medications to be more widely accessible in certain areas.

Third, comorbidity is a consideration (particularly mood and anxiety disorders). One caveat to consider, although, is that successful treatment of eating disorder symptoms may relieve comorbid mood and anxiety. This is especially true for weight restoration and AN. For this reason, when weight restoration is ongoing, watchful waiting to see the extent to which mood and anxiety symptoms resolve is quite defensible. On the other hand, persistent, mood and anxiety syndromes do co-occur with AN, BN, and BED, and these may benefit from medications.

Last is the issue of patient choice. People seeking treatment often have specific views about which treatments they would prefer to receive. Many people prefer psychotherapy, but, for some, medication treatment may feel preferable.

Goals

The general goals of medication treatment deserve careful consideration. In other psychiatric illnesses, various concepts of treatment response are seen. For example, sometimes syndromal remission of the psychopathology is the goal. Examples would probably include major depression or panic disorder. In other instances, reduction of symptoms without full syndromal remission would be the goal; an example would be medication treatment of schizophrenia. Still another possibility would be the goal of preventing recurrence, as could be the case in bipolar illness.

Complicating the consideration of goals of pharmacologic treatment of eating disorders, most psychopharmacology studies in eating disorders have involved acute treatment, typically not lasting beyond 8 or 12 weeks. There is limited work on relapse prevention in AN, which will be reviewed, and one study attempting to look at long-term treatment of BN, but, for the most part, the duration of treatment in the existing literature falls far short of the a typical course of clinical treatment. Given this, longer-term treatment must proceed with little guiding evidence base.

The likely goals of medication use in AN should be symptom reduction, and perhaps as a strategy to facilitate other types of treatments. Abstinence seems a reasonable treatment goal in the treatment of BN and BED, which is seen in a ministry of participants in many published studies. On the other hand, there is some reason to think that this may not usually be full syndromal remission: most studies that have assessed eating behaviors and eating disorder cognitions have found that, when abstinence from binge eating and purging is achieved, significant eating disorder cognitions remain, at least in the short term.

Duration of Treatment

The appropriate duration of medication treatment of eating disorders is unknown and largely untested. A reasonable guide might be the model often used in the treatment of major depression, in which the goal of a year of stability followed by a slow taper with careful monitoring is a reasonable and commonly used clinically strategy.

ANOREXIA NERVOSA

The list of agents that have been tried for the treatment of AN is unusually broad (**Table 1**). This reflects the fact that AN has been largely nonresponsive to medication treatments (and, of course, not highly responsive to other treatments as well, at least in adults). The list includes medications no longer widely used in general psychiatric practice (for example, tricyclic antidepressants or typical antipsychotic medications). Furthermore, it includes medications not easily managed in, or tolerated by, individuals at low weight who are prone to dehydration (for example, lithium[2] or clonidine[3]). Interestingly, tetrahydrocannabinol was examined in a randomized, controlled trial and did not seem to be beneficial.[4] Presently, marijuana-related compounds are increasingly used for many conditions, but it is important to note that the use of tetrahydrocannabinol for AN long predates the recent interest in marijuana as a medical treatment; this should be interpreted as reflecting the challenge inherent in treating AN.

It is worth reviewing several specific medications in this regard. First, there has been substantial interest in the role of altered serotonin neurotransmission in the pathophysiology of AN.[5] In keeping with this interest, several trials have examined the use of fluoxetine. These include acute treatment trials[6] in which treatment does not seem to be beneficial. One might imagine that this represents nutritional lack of serotonin precursors, but Barbarich and colleagues[7] found that co-administration of tryptophan, a precursor to serotonin synthesis, did not potentiate fluoxetine effects. There has also been interest in the use of fluoxetine as a relapse prevention agent. An open trial showed no benefit,[8] but the first large prospective trial suggested some benefit of fluoxetine.[9] Subsequently, a more definitive multicenter trial using

Table 1
Medications studied in blinded, controlled for AN

Positive Trial	Negative Trial
Olanzapine	Pimozide
	Sulpiride
	Cisapride
	Clonidine
	Zinc
	Tetrahydrocannabinol
	Lithium
	Cyproheptadine
	Amitriptyline
	Clomipramine
	Nortriptyline
	Fluoxetine

fluoxetine as a relapse prevention strategy in AN relapse prevention was conducted.[10] This study enrolled 120 participants, who received up to 60 mg of fluoxetine per day for a year after first achieving a body mass index of at least 19. Placebo and active medication did not differ in preventing relapse; thus, it seems that selective serotonin reuptake inhibitors (SSRIs) are not effective for AN. It is possible that there may be selected subgroups that benefit, but these have not been identified in the completed trials.

The second area of recent interest in medication treatment of AN involves atypical antipsychotics. A recent multicenter trial examined the use of olanzapine in acute treatment of AN.[11] This study of 152 people with AN showed about 1 lb per month greater weight gain in the olanzapine group. This benefit may be sufficient to justify the use of olanzapine. In considering these medications, one must consider the potential risks, including tardive dyskinesia and neuroleptic malignant syndrome, versus the potential benefits of accelerated weight restoration. Certainly, patient acceptance of this medication, given its potential for weight gain, is a challenge in using it in this population. Interestingly, Attia[12] have reported that the elevations in lipids and impairments in glucose tolerance seen in other patient populations (for example, those with schizophrenia or bipolar illness), do not seem to occur in people with AN. At this time, it is unclear whether this reflects the unique nutritional status of those with anorexia nervosa, or represents a different metabolic profile in those with AN, suggested by recent work.[13]

BULIMIA NERVOSA

As in AN, many studies have looked at medication treatments for BN over the last few decades. Unlike AN, medications seem to be effective in treating BN (**Box 1**). The first medication approved by the FDA for treatment of an eating disorder was fluoxetine used for treatment of BN.

Early work in this area was often based on alternative conceptualizations of BN causation and maintenance. At one point, anticonvulsants were used extensively, reflecting the possibility that the cause of BN was an underlying seizure disorder.[14] Subsequently, it was argued that BN might be a manifestation of a mood disorder.[15] This led to extensive work with antidepressants. Although BN is no longer thought to be a mood disorder variant, because of the efficacy shown by initial antidepressant studies, this work has continued.

Box 1
Medications shown to have efficacy for BN
Fluoxetine
Fluvoxamine
Citalopram
Sertraline
Amitriptyline
Imipramine
Desipramine
Trazodone
Phenelzine
Topiramate

Two studies of fluoxetine have led it to be the most-often considered medication for BN in the treatment of bulimia nervosa. In this instance, there have been 2 large studies conducted, and these contributed to a great degree to a decision made by the FDA to approve fluoxetine for the treatment of BN. One of these studies compared 60 mg fluoxetine with placebo in 482 people[16] for 16 weeks. The other was a 3-cell design with participants randomized to receive either 60 mg/d of fluoxetine, 20 mg/d of fluoxetine, or placebo.[17] In this study with 387 participants, substantial improvements were seen in binge eating and purging, and substantial rates of abstinence from binge eating at the end of treatment were described. Sixty mg was clearly more effective than 20 mg; 20 mg was more effective than placebo on some outcomes but not others. This has led to the widespread recommendation of fluoxetine as a starting point of pharmacologic treatment of BN. Furthermore, it is led to the recommendation for high-dose (ie, 60 or 80 mg) fluoxetine treatment. In at least one instance, a sequential treatment approach initiated medication treatment with 60 mg/d.[18] In that study, the 60-mg starting dose was actually quite well tolerated. However, it seems likely that some would respond to lower doses if doses were titrated, and that some individuals would be likely not to tolerate 60 mg, so typically clinical practice involves starting at 20 mg with the anticipation that titration to a relatively high dose will likely be necessary.

Alternative Medication Treatments for Bulimia Nervosa

A wide variety of alternative treatments have been studied and been shown to be effective. There is support in the literature for the use of other SSRIs, and they typically represent a second line of treatment. One caveat in this regard, however, is that the FDA has recognized concerns about prolonged QTc in individuals receiving high doses of citalopram.[19] Given the probable need for high doses of SSRIs for good response, this limits citalopram (and perhaps escitalopram) for BN treatment.

There is a remarkably deep literature on the use of tricyclic antidepressants for BN. This spans work using amitriptyline and desipramine, primarily, with several extensive studies examining desipramine.[20–23] Among these, desipramine seems the logical choice. Desipramine has less anticholinergic side effects, less cardiac effects, less sedation, and is less likely to induce weight gain than other tricyclics. Furthermore, there is an ample literature supporting its use in BN. Last, standardized blood levels are available for depression (which one assumes would generalize to the treatment of BN, although this is not fully clear).

Trazodone represents an alternative treatment, supported in other trials, although sedation and orthostasis may limit its use somewhat.[24] Monoamine oxidase (MAO) inhibitors can be used, as noted above.[25,26] Finally, topiramate has been examined in one trial and has been shown to decrease binge eating and purging, although significant weight loss occurred.[27] This may limit its use in BN in patients with a low-normal weight, and certainly in patients with a history of sub-normal weight or AN.

Contraindications

Bupropion is contraindicated in the treatment of BN because of an elevated risk for seizures that was identified in the one study of bupropion that has been conducted in this area.[28] Questions are often raised about whether MAO inhibitors are contraindicated, related to the possibility of dietary violations of a low-tyramine diet leading to hypertensive crises. This has not been observed in clinical trials of MAO inhibitors for BN, and in clinical practice it seems to be rare. On the other hand, the introduction of a low-tyramine diet provides dietary limitations and rules for a group of individuals who generally have an excessive number of dietary rules to begin with, so this is a limitation.

BINGE EATING DISORDER
Treatment Goals

The main treatment goal for BED is cessation of binge eating. The other psychological components of BED enumerated in DSM-5 are also reasonable treatment goals, but tend to receive less emphasis than diminishment or elimination of binge eating. A second treatment goal involves weight loss. This remains a somewhat controversial issue within the eating disorders field, and is sometimes less of a treatment focus for providers. On the other hand, it tends to be at least as important to many individuals with BEDs as the cessation of binge eating itself. It is important to clarify the extent to which this is a treatment goal, and to clearly lay out the expectations the patient may have and the expectations that may be reasonable to achieve based on the existing literature, as these may be quite different.

Agents Studied

Treatment development for BED initially mirrored the path seen in BN. Initial studies examined tricyclic antidepressants and then moved on to SSRIs. Much of this work for a long time has focused on antidepressant medications, and at this point an even wider array of antidepressants has been examined in controlled studies for BED than for BN (**Box 2**). These include trials of fluoxetine,[29] fluvoxamine,[30] citalopram,[31] escitalopram,[32] bupropion,[33] duloxetine,[34] lamotrigine,[35] sertraline,[36] and atomoxetine.[37] Most of these studies have been positive, showing greater decrease in binge eating symptoms and/or greater levels of abstinence in binge eating after treatment in those receiving medications compared with those receiving placebo. An important aspect of these medication trials, however, has been that the major effect has been on binge eating. The overall rates of binge eating tend to decrease fairly markedly, and a significant minority of people receiving medication treatment are abstinent from binge eating at the end of short-term treatment (although, as in BN, little is known about the long-term course). Weight loss with antidepressant medications has not typically been seen, even when major reductions or abstinence from binge eating has been achieved.

| Box 2 |
Medications shown to have efficacy for BED
Fluoxetine
Fluvoxamine
Citalopram
Escitalopram
Sertraline
Duloxetine
Bupropion
Lamotrigine
Topiramate
Zonisamide
Lisdexamfetamine

A new direction in binge eating pharmacotherapy, partially driven by concerns about a need for weight loss, has been the examination of medications that have direct or indirect effects on appetite. For example, the agent fenfluramine, previously used for weight loss but now taken off the market because of concerns about heart valve lesions, was examined and shown to diminish binge eating (although curiously, not to cause weight loss).[38] Subsequently, sibutramine was studied in several trials[39,40] and clearly can diminish binge eating and cause weight loss, but it too has been removed from the market because of concerns about elevated blood pressure. The anticonvulsant agents topiramate[41–43] and zonisamide[44] have also been examined, as each have been noted to diminish appetite; this was seen as a side-effect in many anticonvulsant trials, but in this instance is viewed as a desired treatment effect. Treatment with these agents does lead to significant decreases in BED, and does lead to modest, persisting weight loss; this has been particularly clear in the case of topiramate. There is one longer-term study with topiramate[43] that suggests that there is persisting effect on binge eating symptoms.

Finally, the most recent effort in regard to medication treatments for BED has been a series of studies involving lisdexamfetamine.[45–47] In this regard, several large studies have shown clear evidence of impact on binge eating, with modest impacts on weight. Numerically, the magnitude of clinical response in these studies seems similar to that seen with other BED medication treatments. These studies have led to FDA indication for the use of lisdexamfetamine in the treatment of BED.

AVOIDANT/RESTRICTIVE FOOD INTAKE DISORDER

With the advent of DSM-5, ARFID has received increasing attention. However, behavioral treatments for ARFID in general are only now being worked out,[48] and appropriate medication treatments are not at all clear. Gray and colleagues[49] recently described a case series of 14 individuals receiving mirtazapine (6 as monotherapy, 8 as combination therapy). This study was uncontrolled, so the impacts attributable to mirtazapine treatment are not completely clear, but the authors note that the rate of weight gain exceeded that typically seen in their treatment-as-usual ARFID program. They hypothesize that mirtazapine could be beneficial because it increases appetite, causes weight gain, diminishes nausea and vomiting, and increases rates of gastric emptying.

Clearly, continued medication development in this area is needed. Our understanding of the underlying psychopathology process in ARFID is growing[50] and this may help guide pharmacologic treatment development.

OTHER SPECIFIED FEEDING OR EATING DISORDER

There currently exist no data on medication treatments for OSFED, including subthreshold AN, subthreshold BN, or purging disorder. Clearly development of such treatments is needed; observational studies of people receiving treatment for OSFED suggest that remission rates are relatively limited.[51] This highlights the need for development of new and effective treatments, and certainly raises the possibility that medications may play a role. In clinical practice decisions about medications are commonly made on a symptom-by-symptom basis, assuming that responses are relatively similar to those seen in similar symptom presentations. So, for example, medication strategies seen to be helpful for BN are often used in the treatment of purging disorder. Similarly, what we know about medication treatments for AN is presumed by many clinicians to apply to subthreshold AN.

SUMMARY

Medications, at present, play a limited role in treatment of AN, although there is current interest in the potential utility of atypical antipsychotics. A wide variety of medications, primarily antidepressants, can be beneficial in BN. Antidepressants are also potentially useful for BED symptoms, and medications that suppress appetite can diminish or eliminate binge eating as well. The only 2 FDA-approved medications for eating disorder treatments at present are fluoxetine for BN, and lisdexamfetamine for BED. This remains an area of active research interest, and one in which substantial further development is needed.

REFERENCES

1. Crow SJ, Agras WS, Halmi KA, et al. A cost effectiveness analysis of stepped care treatment for bulimia nervosa. Int J Eat Disord 2013;46(4):302–7.
2. Gross H, Ebert MH, Faden VB, et al. A double-blind trial of delta 9-tetrahydrocannabinol in primary anorexia nervosa. J Clin Psychopharmacol 1983;3(3):165–71.
3. Casper RC, Schlemmer RF Jr, Javaid JI. A placebo-controlled crossover study of oral clonidine in acute anorexia nervosa. Psychiatry Res 1987;20(3):249–60.
4. Gross HA, Ebert MH, Faden VB, et al. A double-blind controlled trial of lithium carbonate primary anorexia nervosa. J Clin Psychopharmacol 1981;1(6): 376–81.
5. Kaye WH, Wierenga CE, Bailer UF, et al. Nothing tastes as good as skinny feels: the neurobiology of anorexia nervosa. Trends Neurosci 2013;36(2):110–20.
6. Attia E, Haiman C, Walsh BT, et al. Does fluoxetine augment the inpatient treatment of anorexia nervosa? Am J Psychiatry 1998;155(4):548–51.
7. Barbarich NC, McConaha CW, Halmi KA, et al. Use of nutritional supplements to increase the efficacy of fluoxetine in the treatment of anorexia nervosa. Int J Eat Disord 2004;35(1):10–5.
8. Strober M, Freeman R, DeAntonio M, et al. Does adjunctive fluoxetine influence the post-hospital course of restrictor-type anorexia nervosa? A 24-month prospective, longitudinal followup and comparison with historical controls. Psychopharmacol Bull 1997;33(3):425–31.
9. Kaye WH, Nagata T, Weltzin TE, et al. Double-blind placebo-controlled administration of fluoxetine in restricting- and restricting-purging-type anorexia nervosa. Biol Psychiatry 2001;49(7):644–52.
10. Walsh BT, Kaplan AS, Attia E, et al. Fluoxetine after weight restoration in anorexia nervosa: a randomized controlled trial. JAMA 2006;295(22):2605–12.
11. Attia E. Presentation at the Eating Disorders Research Society annual meeting. New York: 2016.
12. Attia E. Presented at the Eating Disorder Research Society annual meeting. Sydney (Australia): 2018.
13. Duncan L, Yilmaz Z, Gaspar H, et al. Significant locus and metabolic genetic correlations revealed in genome-wide association study of anorexia nervosa. Am J Psychiatry 2017;174(9):850–8.
14. Wermuth BM, Davis KL, Hollister LE, et al. Phenytoin treatment of the binge-eating syndrome. Am J Psychiatry 1977;134(11):1249–53.
15. Pope HG Jr, Hudson JI. Antidepressant drug therapy for bulimia: current status. J Clin Psychiatry 1986;47(7):339–45.
16. Goldstein DJ, Wilson MG, Thompson VL, et al. Long-term fluoxetine treatment of bulimia nervosa. Fluoxetine Bulimia Nervosa Research Group. Br J Psychiatry 1995;166(5):660–6.

17. FBNC Study Group. Fluoxetine in the treatment of bulimia nervosa. A multicenter, placebo-controlled, double-blind trial. Fluoxetine Bulimia Nervosa Collaborative Study Group. Arch Gen Psychiatry 1992;49(2):139–47.
18. Mitchell JE, Agras WS, Wilson GT, et al. A trial of a relapse prevention strategy in women with bulimia nervosa who respond to cognitive-behavior therapy. Int J Eat Disord 2004;35(4):549–55.
19. U.S. Food and Drug Administration. FDA drug safety communication: revised recommendations for Celexa (citaloprm hydrobromide) related to a potential risk of abnormal heart rhythms with high doses. 2012. Available at: https://www.fda.gov/Drugs/DrugSafety/ucm297391.htm. Accessed December 1, 2018.
20. Barlow J, Blouin J, Blouin A, et al. Treatment of bulimia with desipramine: a double-blind crossover study. Can J Psychiatry 1988;33(2):129–33.
21. Hughes PL, Wells LA, Cunningham CJ, et al. Treating bulimia with desipramine. A double-blind, placebo-controlled study. Arch Gen Psychiatry 1986;43(2):182–6.
22. McCann UD, Agras WS. Successful treatment of nonpurging bulimia nervosa with desipramine: a double-blind, placebo-controlled study. Am J Psychiatry 1990;147(11):1509–13.
23. Walsh BT, Hadigan CM, Devlin MJ, et al. Long-term outcome of antidepressant treatment for bulimia nervosa. Am J Psychiatry 1991;148(9):1206–12.
24. Pope HG Jr, Keck PE Jr, McElroy SL, et al. A placebo-controlled study of trazodone in bulimia nervosa. J Clin Psychopharmacol 1989;9(4):254–9.
25. Kennedy SH, Piran N, Garfinkel PE. Monoamine oxidase inhibitor therapy for anorexia nervosa and bulimia: a preliminary trial of isocarboxazid. J Clin Psychopharmacol 1985;5(5):279–85.
26. Walsh BT, Gladis M, Roose SP, et al. Phenelzine vs. placebo in 50 patients with bulimia. Arch Gen Psychiatry 1988;45(5):471–5.
27. Hoopes SP, Reimherr FW, Hedges DW, et al. Treatment of bulimia nervosa with topiramate in a randomized, double-blind, placebo-controlled trial, part 1: improvement in binge and purge measures. J Clin Psychiatry 2003;64(11):1335–41.
28. Horne RL, Ferguson JM, Pope HG Jr, et al. Treatment of bulimia with bupropion: a multicenter controlled trial. J Clin Psychiatry 1988;49(7):262–6.
29. Arnold LM, McElroy SL, Hudson JI, et al. A placebo-controlled, randomized trial of fluoxetine in the treatment of binge-eating disorder. J Clin Psychiatry 2002;63(11):1028–33.
30. Hudson JI, McElroy SL, Raymond NC, et al. Fluvoxamine in the treatment of binge-eating disorder: a multicenter placebo-controlled, double-blind trial. Am J Psychiatry 1998;155(12):1756–62.
31. Merikangas K, Avenevoli S, Costello J, et al. National comorbidity survey replication adolescent supplement (NCS-A): I. Background and measures. J Am Acad Child Adolesc Psychiatry 2009;48(4):367–9.
32. Guerdjikova AI, McElroy SL, Kotwal R, et al. High-dose escitalopram in the treatment of binge-eating disorder with obesity: a placebo-controlled monotherapy trial. Hum Psychopharmacol 2008;23(1):1–11.
33. White MA, Grilo CM. Bupropion for overweight women with binge-eating disorder: a randomized, double-blind, placebo-controlled trial. J Clin Psychiatry 2013;74(4):400–6.
34. Guerdjikova AI, McElroy SL, Winstanley EL, et al. Duloxetine in the treatment of binge eating disorder with depressive disorders: a placebo-controlled trial. Int J Eat Disord 2012;45(2):281–9.

35. Guerdjikova AI, McElroy SL, Welge JA, et al. Lamotrigine in the treatment of binge-eating disorder with obesity: a randomized, placebo-controlled monotherapy trial. Int Clin Psychopharmacol 2009;24(3):150–8.

36. McElroy SL, Casuto LS, Nelson EB, et al. Placebo-controlled trial of sertraline in the treatment of binge eating disorder. Am J Psychiatry 2000;157(6):1004–6.

37. McElroy SL, Guerdjikova A, Kotwal R, et al. Atomoxetine in the treatment of binge-eating disorder: a randomized placebo-controlled trial. J Clin Psychiatry 2007; 68(3):390–8.

38. Stunkard A, Berkowitz R, Tanrikut C, et al. d-fenfluramine treatment of binge eating disorder. Am J Psychiatry 1996;153(11):1455–9.

39. Appolinario JC, Bacaltchuk J, Sichieri R, et al. A randomized, double-blind, placebo-controlled study of sibutramine in the treatment of binge-eating disorder. Arch Gen Psychiatry 2003;60(11):1109–16.

40. Wilfley DE, Crow SJ, Hudson JI, et al. Efficacy of sibutramine for the treatment of binge eating disorder: a randomized multicenter placebo-controlled double-blind study. Am J Psychiatry 2008;165(1):51–8.

41. McElroy SL, Arnold LM, Shapira NA, et al. Topiramate in the treatment of binge eating disorder associated with obesity: a randomized, placebo-controlled trial. Am J Psychiatry 2003;160(2):255–61.

42. McElroy SL, Hudson JI, Capece JA, et al. Topiramate for the treatment of moderate to severe binge eating disorder associated with obesity: a double-blind, placebo-controlled study. Neuropharmacology 2005;30:S138.

43. McElroy SL, Shapira NA, Arnold LM, et al. Topiramate in the long-term treatment of binge-eating disorder associated with obesity. J Clin Psychiatry 2004;65(11): 1463–9.

44. McElroy SL, Kotwal R, Guerdjikova AI, et al. Zonisamide in the treatment of binge eating disorder with obesity: a randomized controlled trial. J Clin Psychiatry 2006; 67(12):1897–906.

45. Hudson JI, McElroy SL, Ferreira-Cornwell MC, et al. Efficacy of lisdexamfetamine in adults with moderate to severe binge-eating disorder: a randomized clinical trial. JAMA Psychiatry 2017;74(9):903–10.

46. McElroy SL, Hudson J, Ferreira-Cornwell MC, et al. Lisdexamfetamine dimesylate for adults with moderate to severe binge eating disorder: results of two pivotal phase 3 randomized controlled trials. Neuropsychopharmacology 2016;41(5): 1251–60.

47. McElroy SL, Hudson JI, Mitchell JE, et al. Efficacy and safety of lisdexamfetamine for treatment of adults with moderate to severe binge eating disorder: a randomized clinical trial. JAMA Psychiatry 2015;72(3):235–46.

48. Thomas JJ, Wons OB, Eddy KT. Cognitive-behavioral treatment of avoidant/restrictive food intake disorder. Curr Opin Psychiatry 2018;31(6):425–30.

49. Gray E, Chen T, Menzel J, et al. Mirtazapine and weight gain in avoidant and restrictive food intake disorder. J Am Acad Child Adolesc Psychiatry 2018; 57(4):288–9.

50. Thomas JJ, Lawson EA, Micali N, et al. Avoidant/restrictive food intake disorder: a three-dimensional model of neurobiology with implications for etiology and treatment. Curr Psychiatry Rep 2017;19(8):54.

51. Riesco N, Aguera Z, Granero R, et al. Other specified feeding or eating disorders (OSFED): clinical heterogeneity and cognitive-behavioral therapy outcome. Eur Psychiatry 2018;54:109–16.

Medical Complications of Eating Disorders

Medical Complications of Anorexia Nervosa and Bulimia Nervosa

Dennis Gibson, MD[a,b], Cassandra Workman, MD[c],
Philip S. Mehler, MD[a,b,c],*

KEYWORDS

- Medical complications • Eating disorders • Anorexia nervosa • Bulimia nervosa

KEY POINTS

- Anorexia nervosa and bulimia nervosa are multisystem diseases with medical complications affecting all body systems.
- The medical complications of anorexia nervosa are due to malnutrition and weight loss. Additional complications of anorexia nervosa, binge-eating/purging type are due to the frequency and mode of purging behaviors.
- The medical complications of bulimia nervosa are due to the frequency and mode of purging behaviors.

INTRODUCTION

Unlike other psychiatric disorders that do not inherently manifest with somatic complications, eating disorders are multisystem diseases with significant medical complications affecting all body systems. Eating disorders have been noted to have among the highest mortality of all mental health disorders, with mortality in anorexia nervosa (AN) approaching 6% per decade.[1] Although about one-quarter of these deaths in AN are related to suicide, greater than 50% are attributed to medical complications.[1] The purpose of this article is to discuss the medical complications of AN and bulimia nervosa (BN) as well as the recommended interventions. Unless otherwise specified, AN will refer to both AN-R (restricting subtype) and AN-BP (binge/purge subtype).

SKIN

In decreasing order of frequency, the skin manifestations of AN include xerosis (dry skin), hypertrichosis lanuginosa (lanugo hair), telogen effluvium (hair loss), nail fragility,

Disclosure Statement: None of the authors have any disclosures to declare.
a ACUTE @ Denver Health, 777 Bannock Street, Denver, CO 80204, USA; b Department of Medicine, University of Colorado School of Medicine, 13001 E 17th Pl, Aurora, CO, 80045, USA; c Eating Recovery Center, 7351 East Lowry Boulevard, Suite 200, Denver, CO 80230, USA
* Corresponding author.
E-mail address: Philip.mehler@dhha.org

and acrocyanosis.[2–4] Purpura and easy bruisability are also found in AN, related to thrombocytopenia.[3] These skin changes are in part an expected physiologic adaption to the malnutrition and associated hypothermia commonly present in individuals with eating disorders.[5] Lanugo presents as fine, minimally pigmented hairs mostly on the face, back, or abdomen.[6] It is not a sign of virilization and likely serves as a heat-conserving mechanism.[2,3] Acrocyanosis is a condition of skin arteriole constriction and venous dilatation of unknown cause. It has been hypothesized to serve as an energy-saving mechanism.[7] Xerosis likely develops secondary to various nutrient deficiencies as well as reduced sebaceous gland secretion and altered composition of the secreted sebum.[3,6,8] Telogen effluvium manifests as a diffuse pattern of hair loss due to an increased number of hairs in the telogen phase, the resting phase when hair loss occurs.[3,6] Individuals who engage in purging via self-induced vomiting may manifest with Russell sign, thickening of the skin over dorsal surface of the knuckles, and is considered a pathognomonic sign for AN-BP and BN.[8] Male patients with AN may be less prone to develop lanugo and may present with a higher frequency of striae distensae (stretch marks).[8,9] All these conditions improve with weight restoration and cessation of vomiting.

HEAD, EARS, EYES, NOSE, THROAT

Lagophthalmos, the inability to fully close the eyelids, leads to symptoms of eye irritation due to ocular surface drying. Lagophthalmos is presumed to be secondary to orbital fat wasting[10] and is proportional to the extent of weight loss. It is treated with lubrication and weight restoration. Autophonia, the hyperperception of one's own voice and breathing, is another occurrence in severe AN. It is thought to be secondary to loss of fatty tissue surrounding the eustachian tube. Improvement is seen with weight restoration.[11,12] Oropharyngeal dysphagia is a relatively common symptom in this population as well, due to weakness of the swallowing muscles.[13,14] Dysphagia can be well managed in consultation with a speech therapist and with dietary modification leading to strengthening of the swallowing muscles.[13,15]

Complications specific to those who engage in self-induced vomiting include dental erosion of the lingual surface of the teeth known as perimylolysis, increased incidence of dental caries, and sialadenosis, a swelling of the major salivary glands, including the parotid gland, often occurring a few days after purging ceases.[16] Perimylolysis and dental caries seem to develop as a result of food choices, changes in salivary composition, and increased contact of gastric acid with the teeth as a result of vomiting.[3] Sialadenosis can be treated with sialagogues (ie, hard candies such as lemon drops or LifeSavers) to encourage saliva production, heating pads, and anti-inflammatory medications; rarely, pilocarpine may be required for refractory cases.[17] Subconjunctival hemorrhage and epistaxis can also develop as a result of forceful retching.

PULMONARY

The lungs are relatively spared compared with the other body systems. However, there are case reports of spontaneous pneumothorax, pneumomediastinum, and the pulmonary function changes of obstructive lung disease.[14,18–20] Development of pneumomediastinum appears to be secondary to nontraumatic alveolar rupture and not secondary to esophageal perforation. Hence, purging does not appear to increase the risk of spontaneous pneumothorax. Supportive care seems to be adequate in most cases, although chest tube intervention may occasionally be warranted. Aspiration pneumonia also occurs with increased frequency in those with AN and BN due to either oropharyngeal weakness or purging via emesis.[13]

CARDIAC

Sudden cardiac death is a potential cause of the high mortality in those with eating disorders. Sudden cardiac death can be attributed to various functional and structural causes, including myocardial scarring and cardiac atrophy,[21,22] as well as various cardiac arrhythmias. The impact of QT dispersion (inter-lead QT variability on electrocardiogram) toward sudden death and predisposition to unstable arrhythmias seems likely, although medications and duration of disease may be a further influence.[23–27] However, QT prolongation is not inherit to AN or BN, and when present, should result in a search for secondary causes of QT prolongation, such as electrolyte derangements and offending medications.

Other common cardiac manifestations of AN include mitral valve prolapse and pericardial effusion. Mitral valve prolapse occurs in individuals with AN and is related to changes in left ventricular dimensions causing laxity of the mitral valve.[28,29] Pericardial effusion also develops in about one-third of individuals with AN, is of unclear cause, and correlates with the level of malnutrition.[30] Both of these conditions are generally reversible with weight restoration.[30,31]

The most common clinical findings include sinus bradycardia and hypotension. Sinus bradycardia is a nearly universal finding in AN,[32] likely a manifestation of increased vagal tone.[33] Junctional rhythms and other bradyarrhythmias will occasionally develop as well.[34] Patients with marked bradycardia (pulse <35 beats/min) should be monitored with telemetry, but no other intervention or use of a pacemaker is generally required. Bradycardia generally resolves with adequate weight restoration.

Those with AN-BP and BN may be at increased risk for arrhythmias due to electrolyte imbalance. These electrolyte and acid base disorders, as a result of purging behaviors, are likely the cause of the elevated mortality in AN-BP relative to AN-R, and in BN.[35] A cardiomyopathy may also develop if individuals used an excessive amount of Ipecac as a form of purging, or in some cases, as a result of chronic malnutrition in the absences of Ipecac use.[36]

GASTROINTESTINAL

Gastrointestinal (GI) complaints of bloating, early satiety, abdominal discomfort, nausea, and constipation are commonly reported in this population. Many of these symptoms are likely the result of slowed GI motility, which is a common finding in those with AN.[37,38] This diminished motility tends to normalize with weight restoration.[39–41] Gastric-emptying studies are rarely needed for diagnosis of gastroparesis given the near universal finding of prolonged gastric emptying as the severity of weight loss increases; furthermore, gastric emptying times do not correlate well with reported symptoms,[42] suggesting a functional component to these symptoms in AN and BN as well.[42,43] It is unclear if there is a higher incidence of pancreatitis that would contribute to these symptoms, although several potential mechanisms could be postulated regarding an increased risk for those with eating disorders.[44] The constipation and associated straining along with stimulant laxative abuse predispose to development of rectal prolapse.[45] Patient education regarding normalization of gastric and intestinal motility, and thus improvement in abdominal discomfort, bloating, and constipation, can be expected with weight restoration. Prokinetic or motility agents, such as metoclopramide, and osmotic agents, such as polyethylene glycol, are first-line pharmacologic treatments for gastroparesis and constipation, respectively, and may be required temporarily during early refeeding. However, metoclopramide should be used at lower doses to minimize the risk for potential adverse effects of tardive dyskinesia and QT prolongation. Macrolide antibiotics may also be tried, cautiously, for symptoms of delayed gastric emptying.

Superior mesenteric artery (SMA) syndrome is a less frequent cause of abdominal pain and emesis in AN. The true prevalence of this condition in AN is unknown, and weight loss is the greatest risk factor leading to its development.[46] As extent of malnutrition increases, the fat pad that normally supports the SMA is lost, causing its medial migration and resultant total or incomplete compression of the duodenum between the SMA and the aorta. Surgery is not recommended as a first-line treatment because weight restoration, using a soft or liquid oral diet or placement of a feeding tube and bypassing the mechanical obstruction, is successful in most cases.[47] Computed tomographic scan can provide anatomic diagnosis, but upper GI series provides a more functional diagnosis. SMA syndrome also predisposes to the rarely encountered gastric dilatation.[48] Gastric dilatation can be diagnosed with a plain abdominal radiograph and should be treated with nasogastric suction as well as a surgical consult given the increased risk for vascular insufficiency, gastric necrosis, and perforation.

Individuals with AN-BP and BN are at increased risk for esophageal complications due to reflux of gastric acid through the weakened lower esophageal sphincter as a result of purging. A higher incidence of gastroesophageal reflux is reported in BN,[49,50] which may further contribute to serious complications, such as esophageal adenocarcinoma.[51] However, endoscopic findings in those reporting reflux seem to be noted less frequently than expected,[52] suggesting there may be a functional component.[50] Individuals may also develop Mallory-Weiss tears and/or esophageal rupture due to recurrent vomiting. A trial of H2 antagonists and/or proton pump inhibitors along with cessation of purging is the recommended treatment of acid reflux with consideration of an upper endoscopy.

Those engaging in abuse of stimulant laxatives may be at risk for cathartic colon syndrome. Although speculative as to whether this condition develops with currently available stimulant laxatives, this condition is likely due to damage to the gut nerve plexus, creating a colon that is incapable of peristalsis and the propagation of fecal material.[53] It is recommended that stimulant laxatives be discontinued for this reason. A harmless black discoloration of the colon, known as melanosis coli, can also develop with chronic laxative abuse.

HEPATIC

Abnormal liver function tests (aspartate aminotransferase/alanine aminotransferase [AST/ALT]) are a frequent manifestation of both starvation and refeeding in those with eating disorders. Starvation hepatitis is increasingly common with greater weight loss, normalizes with weight restoration, and is not usually associated with elevated bilirubin or alkaline phosphatase.[54] It is thought to be due to autophagy.[55] Abnormal elevations in the AST/ALT can also develop as a result of refeeding, causing steatotic changes.[56] Treatment of refeeding hepatitis can require a decrease in the daily caloric intake and/or carbohydrate intake to improve the inflammatory changes. Ultrasound can differentiate these 2 conditions if diagnosis is in question, with normal findings in starvation but with echogenic changes in refeeding.

HEMATOLOGIC/IMMUNOLOGIC

Abnormalities in the complete blood count of patients with AN are commonly seen and may mimic other severe hematological diseases.[57] Anemia, leukopenia, neutropenia, and, occasionally, thrombocytopenia can be seen, with a certain subset of patients having deficiencies in all 3 cell lines as weight loss becomes more severe. The incidence of anemia, leukopenia, neutropenia, and thrombocytopenia has been stud- ied in a community sample of both outpatient adolescents and severely ill adult pa- tients. Age was inversely related to these changes, with younger patients having a higher proportion of cytopenias.[58] Rates of leukopenia ranged from being present in 22% to 79% of patients and anemia in 22% to 83%, and thrombocytopenia was the least frequent.[59,60] In the sickest population, pancytopenia was found in 23% of patients. The most notable determinants of severity of these cytopenias were related to age and body mass index (BMI), with younger populations and lower BMI individ- uals having the highest incidence. Interestingly, none of these abnormalities seemed to be due to a deficiency in iron, vitamin B12, or folate, and the investigators recom- mended not routinely testing for these deficiencies.[60] The purported mechanism of diminished cell production likely involves decreased bone marrow cellularity and gelatinous marrow transformation.[61] In addition, despite a marked reduction in the white blood cell count, most studies do not show an increase in infection risk in this population.[62] These changes improve with weight restoration and improvement in nutrition, making the use of growth factors unnecessary. Thus, complete blood counts should be monitored when evaluating a patient with AN, and the severity of the counts may give an indication of the severity of the disease, but do not typically require any special precautions or treatments.

NEUROMUSCULOSKELETAL

Patients with AN develop significant muscular weakness and deconditioning, at least partially because of a proximal myopathy with type 2 muscle fiber atrophy that im- proves with weight restoration.[63,64] Neurologic changes in AN include diffuse atrophy of gray and white matter.[65] These neurologic changes are associated with various def- icits on neuropsychological testing that are also found in BN, worsening with greater levels of malnutrition.[66] Although the brain atrophy appears to mostly normalize with weight restoration,[65] the cognitive deficits do not necessarily normalize with weight restoration. It is unclear if these persisting deficits are trait characteristics of the illness, perhaps contributing to development of the eating disorder, or if they are irreversible neurologic deficits developing secondary to the malnutrition.[67,68]

ENDOCRINE

Multiple endocrine dysregulations develop in those with eating disorders, likely as physiologic adaptive mechanisms in response to the extreme starvation. Hypoglyce- mia is frequently observed because of depleted glycogen stores and lack of substrates for gluconeogenesis, with increased frequency as severity of malnutri- tion increases. Hypoglycemia is a common cause of sudden death in AN. The hypothalamic-pituitary-thyroid (HPT) axis is dysregulated in AN with low T3, low T4, and normal thyrotropin.[69] Although a similar pattern is found in malnutrition, weight loss is unlikely the sole cause for these findings given a dysregulated HPT axis is also found in normal weight individuals with BN.[70] Reduced estrogens and an- drogens are often found in this population as a result of decreased and dysregulated gonadotropin-releasing hormone pulsatility and a reversion to a prepubertal state, contributing to hypothalamic amenorrhea.[71] This dysregulated gonadal axis is a result of leptin deficiency that is found in both AN and BN.[72,73] The hypothalamic- pituitary-adrenal axis is dysregulated as well with the finding of increased cortisol levels.[74] This hypercortisolemia increases gluconeogenesis and provides nutrients vital to organ function but may also contribute to a centripetal fat distribution during refeeding, mood-related symptoms, an increased risk of gastric ulcer, and an increased risk of osteoporosis.[75] Growth hormone resistance is also a common finding in AN, contributing to decreased insulinlike growth factor 1 levels and further contributing to the low-bone-mineral density frequently found in this population.[76] Growth hormone resistance may partially develop as a consequence of the lipolytic effects of this hormone.[76] These dysregulated hormonal pathways tend to normalize with weight restoration,[74,76] with the possible exception of bone disease. In addition, fertility is generally restored after recovery from the eating disorder,[77] although active AN can predispose to an increased risk for unplanned pregnancy due to ovulation in the absence of menses.[78] An active eating disorder may also lead to negative birth outcomes, including an increased risk of small-for-gestational-age births and an increased risk of miscarriages.[79] In addition to the decreased leptin levels, other changes in appetite-regulating hormones, including increased ghrelin, peptide YY, and relatively increased adiponectin, have all been described in AN.[80–82]

Low bone density, defined as a z score less than -1 for the diagnosis of osteopenia and less than -2.5 defined as osteoporosis, is common in patients with AN and can be very detrimental to patients long after they recover. This bone disease is thought to be related to several disruptions in the hypothalamic-hypogonadal axis. Because of the patient's inadequate calorie intake, nonessential functions of the body begin to be suppressed or even shut down. Patients with anorexia have significant reductions in serum levels of estrogen and progesterone.[83] Reduced sex hormones contribute to a decrease of bone formation and an increase in bone resorption, leading to the state of reduced bone density.[84] This state of uncoupling is responsible for the severity of bone disease, notwithstanding the often young age of these patients. Misra and colleagues[59] found, in a cohort of 60 adolescent outpatients with AN, that 41% of the patients had osteopenia and osteoporosis. Other studies show as high as an 85% incidence of low bone density as defined by a z score of less than -1.[85] Duration of illness, age, and nadir BMI have been shown to be a significant factor in the severity of bone disease.[86,87] In addition, these lower bone densities lead to a higher long-term incidence of fractures. Many of these patients, in addition to restriction, turn to compulsive exercise as a manifestation of anxiety or method of caloric burning. As opposed to postmenopausal women wherein exercise is beneficial for improving bone density, exercise in these patients is detrimental to bone mineral density.[85] Treatment should be focused on weight restoration because studies have shown that weight restoration will lead to improvement in bone mineral density.[88] Other medications, such as bisphosphonates, teriparatide, and others, have been used, but no definite guidelines currently exist.[89] There are, however, randomized controlled trials that support the judicious use of bisphosphonates, teriparatide, and transdermal estrogen in patients with AN.[83,90] Although transdermal estrogen has been shown to be effective, oral contraceptives (OCPs) and oral estrogen replacement have not been found to be effective, and furthermore, the withdrawal bleed from OCPs can lead to a false sense of recovery in patients.

RENAL AND ELECTROLYTES

Recurrent purging with secondary development of hypokalemia can predispose to hypokalemic nephropathy in AN-BP and BN.[91] The true incidence of this condition in those engaging in purging is unknown, but when it occurs, it can result in end-stage renal disease and the need for hemodialysis.

Individuals with AN-BP and BN who engage in frequent purging often develop electrolyte abnormalities along with excessive weight gain after the abrupt cessation of the excessive purging behavior. This condition, known as pseudo-Bartter syndrome, tends to develop because of sustained increases in release of aldosterone as a result of chronic intravascular depletion, to reduce the risk of syncope, which in turn leads to sodium and water retention along with metabolic alkalosis and hypokalemia.[92] Pseudo-Bartter syndrome should be treated with gentle fluid resuscitation and early initiation of an aldosterone antagonist, such as spironolactone.[93]

Hypophosphatemia during refeeding is one of the most dangerous complications that can develop in AN. Increased weight loss is one of the strongest predictors for development of hypophosphatemia,[94] due to depleted total body phosphorous and further shifting of phosphorous intracellularly with refeeding. Phosphorous should be carefully monitored during refeeding and corrected with oral and, in more severe cases, intravenous supplementation.

Of note, electrolytes are usually normal in those primarily restricting food intake, but hypokalemia and metabolic alkalosis with the potential for acid-base disturbances are a frequent manifestation in BN and AN-BP.[95] Hyponatremia is occasionally seen in patients with AN, most often because of diminished ability for free water clearance from an abnormal solute load in the urine.[96] Hypovolemia can also be an additional cause for development of hyponatremia. Syndrome of inappropriate antidiuretic hormone does not appear to be a common cause of hyponatremia in this population. Less commonly, hypernatremia can also occur as the result of diminished fluid intake or neurogenic diabetes insipidus.[97]

SUMMARY

In summary, the medical complications of AN are generally due to malnutrition and weight loss and their associated physiologic compensations. The complications of purging are due to the frequency and mode of these behaviors. Most medical comorbidities in eating disorders are effectively treated with nutritional rehabilitation and weight restoration, along with cessation of the purging behaviors.

REFERENCES

1. Sullivan P. Mortality in anorexia nervosa. Am J Psychiatry 1995;152(7):1073–4.
2. Glorio R, Allevato M, De Pablo A, et al. Prevalence of cutaneous manifestations in 200 patients with eating disorders. Int J Dermatol 2000;39:348–53.
3. Strumia R. Eating disorders and the skin. Clin Dermatol 2013;31:80–5.
4. Bhanji S, Mattingly D. Acrocyanosis in anorexia nervosa. Postgrad Med J 1991; 67:33–5.
5. Swenne I, Engstrom I. Medical assessment of adolescent girls with eating disorders: an evaluation of symptoms and signs of starvation. Acta Paediatr 2005;94: 1363–71.
6. Tyler I, Wiseman MC, Crawford RI, et al. Cutaneous manifestations of eating disorders. J Cutan Med Surg 2002;6(4):345–53.
7. Freyschuss U, Fohlin L, Thoren C. Temperature regulation in anorexia nervosa. Acta Paediatr Scand 1978;67:225–8.
8. Strumia R. Dermatologic signs in patients with eating disorders. Am J Clin Dermatol 2005;6(3):165–73.
9. Strumia R, Manzato E, Gualandi M. Cutaneous manifestations in male anorexia nervosa: four cases. Acta Derm Venereol 2003;83(6):464–5.
10. Gaudiani JL, Braverman JM, Mascolo M, et al. Ophthalmic changes in severe anorexia nervosa: A case series. Int J Eat Disord 2012;45(5):719–21.
11. Karwautz A, Hafferl A, Ungar D, et al. Patulous Eustachian tube in a case of adolescent anorexia nervosa. Int J Eat Disord 1999;25(3):353–5.

12. Godbole M, Key A. Autophonia in anorexia nervosa. Int J Eat Disord 2010;43: 480–2.

13. Holmes SRM, Sabel AL, Guadiani JL, et al. Prevalence and management of oropharyngeal dysphagia in patients with severe anorexia nervosa: a large retrospective review. Int J Eat Disord 2016;49(2):159–66.

14. Lee KJ, Yun HK, Park IN. Spontaneous pneumomediastinum: an unusual pulmonary complication in anorexia nervosa. Tuberc Respir Dis (Seoul) 2015; 78:360–2.

15. Holmes SRM, Gudridge TA, Gaudiani JL, et al. Dysphagia in severe anorexia nervosa: a case report. Int J Eat Disord 2012;45:463–6.

16. Vavrina J, Muller W, Gebbers JO. Enlargement of salivary glands in bulimia. J Laryngol Otol 1994;108:516–8.

17. Mehler PS, Wallace JA. Sialadenosis in bulimia. A new treatment. Arch Otolaryngol 1993;119:787–8.

18. Jensen VM, Stoving RK, Andersen PE. Anorexia nervosa with massive pulmonary air leak and extraordinary propagation. Int J Eat Disord 2017;50:451–3.

19. Lin LY, Kwok CF, Tang KT, et al. Diffuse soft tissue emphysema in anorexia nervosa: a case report. Int J Eat Disord 2005;38:277–80.

20. Gardenghi GG, Boni E, Todisco P, et al. Respiratory function in patients with stable anorexia nervosa. Chest 2009;136:1356–63.

21. Lamzabi I, Syed S, Reddy VB, et al. Myocardial changes in a patient with anorexia nervosa: a case report and review of literature. Am J Clin Pathol 2015; 143:734–7.

22. Oflaz S, Yucel B, Oz F, et al. Assessment of myocardial damage by cardiac MRI in patients with anorexia nervosa. Int J Eat Disord 2013;46:862–6.

23. Nahshoni E, Weizman A, Yaroslavsky A, et al. Alterations in QT dispersion in the surface electrocardiogram of female adolescents diagnosed with restricting-type anorexia nervosa. J Psychosom Res 2007;62(4):469–72.

24. Krantz MJ, Donahoo WT, Melanson EL, et al. QT interval dispersion and resting metabolic rate in chronic anorexia nervosa. Int J Eat Disord 2005;37:166–70.

25. Nussinovitch M, Gur E, Kaminer K, et al. QT variability among weight-restored patients with anorexia nervosa. Gen Hosp Psychiatry 2012;34:62–5.

26. Nahshoni E, Yaroslavsky A, Varticovschi P, et al. Alterations in QT dispersion in the surface electrocardiogram of female adolescent inpatients diagnosed with bulimia nervosa. Compr Psychiatry 2010;51(4):406–11.

27. Bomba M, Tremolizzo L, Corbetta F, et al. QT interval and dispersion in drug-free anorexia nervosa adolescents: a case control study. Eur Child Adolesc Psychiatry 2018;27:861–6.

28. De Simone G, Scalfi L, Galderisi M, et al. Cardiac abnormalities in young women with anorexia nervosa. Br Heart J 1994;71:287–92.

29. Meyers DG, Starke H, Pearson PH, et al. Leaflet to left ventricular size disproportion and prolapse of structurally normal mitral valve in anorexia nervosa. Am J Cardiol 1987;60(10):911–4.

30. Kastner S, Salbach-Andrae H, Renneberg B, et al. Echocardiographic findings in adolescents with anorexia nervosa at beginning of treatment and after weight recovery. Eur Child Adolesc Psychiatry 2012;21:15–21.

31. Olivares JL, Vazquez M, Fleta J, et al. Cardiac findings in adolescents with anorexia nervosa at diagnosis and after weight restoration. Eur J Pediatr 2005; 164:383–6.

32. Yahalom M, Spitz M, Sandler L, et al. The significance of bradycardia in anorexia nervosa. Int J Angiol 2013;22(2):83–94.

33. Romano C, Chinali M, Pasanisi F, et al. Reduced hemodynamic load and cardiac hypotrophy in patients with anorexia nervosa. Am J Clin Nutr 2003;77(2):308–12.
34. Krantz MJ, Gaudiani JL, Johnson VW, et al. Exercise electrocardiography extinguishes persistent junctional rhythm in a patient with severe anorexia nervosa. Cardiology 2011;120:217–20.
35. Crow SJ, Peterson CB, Swanson SA, et al. Increased mortality in bulimia nervosa and other eating disorders. Am J Psychiatry 2009;166(12):1342–6.
36. Ho PC, Dweik R, Cohen MC. Rapidly reversible cardiomyopathy associated with chronic ipecac ingestion. Clin Cardiol 1998;21:780–3.
37. Stacher G. Oesophageal and gastric motility disorders in patients categorised as having primary anorexia nervosa. Gut 1986;27:1120–6.
38. Kamal J, Chami T, Andersen A, et al. Delayed gastrointestinal transit times in anorexia nervosa and bulimia nervosa. Gastroenterology 1991;101:1320–4.
39. Rigaud D, Bedig G, Merrouche M, et al. Delayed gastric emptying in anorexia nervosa is improved by completion of a renutrition program. Dig Dis Sci 1988;33:919–25.
40. Chun AB, Sokol MS, Kaye WH, et al. Colonic and anorectal function in constipated patients with anorexia nervosa. Am J Gastroenterol 1997;92:1879–83.
41. Martinez-Olmos MA, Peino R, Prieto-Tenreiro A, et al. Intestinal absorption and pancreatic function are preserved in anorexia nervosa patients in both a severely malnourished state and after recovery. Eur Eat Disord Rev 2013;21(3):247–51.
42. Perez ME, Coley B, Crandall W, et al. Effect of nutritional rehabilitation on gastric motility and somatization in adolescents with anorexia. J Pediatr 2013;163(3):867–72.
43. Abraham S, Kellow J. Exploring eating disorder quality of life and functional gastrointestinal disorders among eating disorder patients. J Psychosom Res 2011;70(4):372–7.
44. Morris LG, Stephenson KE, Herring S, et al. Recurrent acute pancreatitis in anorexia and bulimia. JOP 2004;5:231–4.
45. Mitchell N, Norris ML. Rectal prolapse associated with anorexia nervosa: a case report and review of the literature. J Eat Disord 2013;1:39.
46. Welsch T, Buchler MW, Kienle P. Recalling superior mesenteric artery syndrome. Dig Surg 2007;24:149–56.
47. Lee TH, Lee JS, Jo Y, et al. Superior mesenteric artery syndrome: Where do we stand today? J Gastrointest Surg 2012;16(12):2203–11.
48. Mascolo M, Dee E, Townsend R, et al. Severe gastric dilatation due to superior mesenteric artery syndrome in anorexia nervosa. Int J Eat Disord 2015;48:532–4.
49. Winstead N, Willard S. Gastrointestinal complaints in patients with eating disorders. J Clin Gastroenterol 2006;40:678–82.
50. Boyd C, Abraham S, Kellow J. Psychological features are important predictors of functional gastrointestinal disorders in patients with eating disorders. Scand J Gastroenterol 2005;40:929–35.
51. Denholm M, Jankowski J. Gastroesophageal reflux disease and bulimia nervosa—a review of the literature. Dis Esophagus 2011;24:79–85.
52. Kiss A, Wiesnagrotzki S, Abatzi T, et al. Upper gastrointestinal endoscopy findings in patients with long-standing bulimi nervosa. Gastrointest Endosc 1989;35:516–8.
53. Smith B. Pathology of cathartic colon. Proc R Soc Med 1972;65(3):288.
54. Rosen E, Sabel AL, Brinton JT, et al. Liver dysfunction in patients with severe anorexia nervosa. Int J Eat Disord 2016;49(2):151–8.

55. Kheloufi M, Boulanger CM, Durand F, et al. Liver autophagy in anorexia nervosa and acute liver injury. Biomed Res Int 2014;2014:701064.

56. Narayanan V, Gaudiani JL, Harris RH, et al. Liver function test abnormalities in anorexia nervosa—cause or effect. Int J Eat Disord 2010;43:378–81.

57. Hutter G, Ganepola S, Hofmann WK. The hematology of anorexia nervosa. Int J Eat Disord 2009;42:293–300.

58. Gaudiani JL, Briton JT, Sabel AL, et al. Medical outcomes for adults hospitalized with severe anorexia nervosa: an analysis by age group. Int J Eat Disord 2016; 49(4):378–85.

59. Misra M, Aggarwal A, Miller KK, et al. Effects of anorexia nervosa on clinical, hematologic, biochemical, and bone density parameters in community-dwelling adolescent girls. Pediatrics 2004;114:1574–83.

60. Sabel AL, Gaudiani JL, Statland B, et al. Hematological abnormalities in severe anorexia nervosa. Ann Hematol 2013;92:605–13.

61. Abella E, Feliu E, Granada I, et al. Bone marrow changes in anorexia nervosa are correlated with the amount of weight loss and not with other clinical findings. Am J Clin Pathol 2002;118:582–8.

62. Bowers TK, Eckert E. Leukopenia in anorexia nervosa: Lack of increased risk of infection. Arch Intern Med 1978;138:1520–3.

63. McLoughlin DM, Spargo E, Wassif WS, et al. Structural and functional changes in skeletal muscle in anorexia nervosa. Acta Neuropathol 1998;95:632–40.

64. McLoughlin DM, Wassif WS, Morton J, et al. Metabolic abnormalities associated with skeletal myopathy in severe anorexia nervosa. Nutrition 2000;16: 192–6.

65. Seitz J, Buhren K, von Polier GG, et al. Morphological changes in the brain of acutely ill and weight-recovered patients with anorexia nervosa: a meta-analysis and qualitative review. Z Kinder Jugendpsychiatr Psychother 2014; 42(1):7–18.

66. Cand SW, Indredavik MS, Lydersen S, et al. Neuropsychological function in patients with anorexia or bulimia nervosa. Int J Eat Disord 2015;48:397–405.

67. Bosanac P, Kurlender S, Stojanovska L, et al. Neuropsychological study of underweight and "weight-recovered" anorexia nervosa compared with bulimia nervosa and normal controls. Int J Eat Disord 2007;40:613–21.

68. Nikendei C, Funiok C, Pfuller U, et al. Memory performance in acute and weight-restored anorexia nervosa patients. Psychol Med 2011;41:829–38.

69. Bannai C, Kuzuya N, Koide Y, et al. Assessment of the relationship between serum thyroid hormone levels and peripheral metabolism in patients with anorexia nervosa. Endocrinol Jpn 1988;35:455–62.

70. Gwirtsman HE, Roy Byrne P, Yager J, et al. Neuroendocrine abnormalities in bulimia. Am J Psychiatry 1983;140:559–63.

71. Boyar RM, Katz J, Finkelstein JW, et al. Anorexia nervosa—immaturity of the 24-hour luteinizing hormone secretory pattern. N Engl J Med 1974;291:861–5.

72. Mehler PS, Eckel RH, Donahoo WT. Leptin levels in restricting and purging anorectics. Int J Eat Disord 1999;26(2):189–94.

73. Brewerton TD, Lesem MD, Kennedy A, et al. Reduced plasma leptin concentrations in bulimia nervosa. Psychoneuroendocrinology 2000;25(7):649–58.

74. Monteleone AM, Monteleone P, Serino I, et al. Underweight subjects with anorexia nervosa have an enhanced salivary cortisol response not seen in weight restored subjects with anorexia nervosa. Psychoneuroendocrinology 2016;70: 118–21.

75. Miller KK. Endocrine dysregulation in anorexia nervosa update. J Clin Endocrinol Metab 2011;96(10):2939–49.
76. Misra M, Miller KK, Bjornson J, et al. Alterations in growth hormone secretory dynamics in adolescent girls with anorexia nervosa and effects on bone metabolism. J Clin Endocrinol 2003;88:5615–23.
77. Wentz E, Gillberg IC, Anckarsater H, et al. Reproduction and offspring status 18 years after teenage-onset anorexia nervosa—A controlled community-based study. Int J Eat Disord 2009;42(6):483–91.
78. Bulik CM, Hoffman ER, von Holle A, et al. Unplanned pregnancy in women with anorexia nervosa. Obstet Gynecol 2010;116:1136–40.
79. Linna MS, Raevuori A, Haukka J, et al. Pregnancy, obstetric, and perinatal health outcomes in eating disorders. Am J Obstet Gynecol 2014;211:392 e1–8.
80. Otto B, Cuntz U, Fruehauf E, et al. Weight gain decreases elevated plasma ghrelin concentrations of patients with anorexia nervosa. Eur J Endocrinol 2001;145: 669–73.
81. Misra M, Miller KK, Tsai P, et al. Elevated peptide YY levels in adolescent girls with anorexia nervosa. J Clin Endocrinol Metab 2006;91(3):1027–33.
82. Khalil RB, Hachem CE. Adiponectin in eating disorders. Eat Weight Disord 2014; 19(1):3–10.
83. Fazeli PK, Klibanski A. Anorexia nervosa and bone metabolism. Bone 2014;66: 39–45.
84. Viapiana O, Gatti D, Grave RD, et al. Marked increases in bone mineral density and biochemical markers of bone turnover in patients with anorexia nervosa gaining weight. Bone 2007;40:1073–7.
85. Miller KK, Grinspoon SK, Ciampa J, et al. Medical findings in outpatients with anorexia nervosa. Arch Intern Med 2005;165(5):561–6.
86. Solmi M, Veronese MN, Correl CU, et al. Bone mineral density, osteoporosis and fractures among people with eating disorders: a systematic review and meta-analysis. Acta Psychiatr Scand 2016;133:341–51.
87. Robinson L, Aldreidge V, Clark EM, et al. A systematic review and meta-analysis of the association between eating disorders and bone density. Osteoporos Int 2016;7(6):1953–66.
88. Ghoch ME, Gatti D, Calugi S, et al. The association between weight gain/restoration and bone mineral density in adolescents with anorexia nervosa: a systematic review. Nutrients 2016;8(12):769.
89. Drabkin A, Rothman MS, Wassenaar E, et al. Assessment and clinical management of bone disease in adults with eating disorders: a review. J Eat Disord 2017;5:42.
90. Golden NH, Iglesias EA, Jacobson MS, et al. Alendronate for the treatment of osteopenia in anorexia nervosa: a randomized, double-blind, placebo-controlled trial. J Clin Endocrinol Metab 2005;90(6):3179–85.
91. Chih-chia L, Hung-Chieh Y. Hypokalemic nephropathy in anorexia nervosa. CMAJ 2011;183(11):E761.
92. Bahia A, Mascolo M, Gaudiani JL, et al. PseudoBartter syndrome in eating disorders. Int J Eat Disord 2012;45:150–3.
93. Mehler PS. Eating disorders. N Engl J Med 1999;341:614–6.
94. Brown CA, Sabel AL, Gaudiani JL, et al. Predictors of hypophosphatemia during refeeding of patients with severe anorexia nervosa. Int J Eat Disord 2015;48: 898–904.

95. Mehler PS, Blalock DV, Waldeen K, et al. Medical findings in 1,026 consecutive adult inpatient-residential eating disordered patients. Int J Eat Disord 2018; 51(4):305–13.
96. Bahia A, Chu ES, Mehler PS. Polydipsia and hyponatremia in a woman with anorexia nervosa. Int J Eat Disord 2011;44:186–8.
97. Hayashida M, Inagaki T, Horiguchi J. Anorexia nervosa and diabetes insipidus in pregnancy. Prog Neuropsychopharmacol Biol Psychiatry 2011;35:297–8.

Medical Complications of Binge Eating Disorder

Elizabeth Wassenaar, MS, MD[a],*, Julie Friedman, PhD[b], Philip S. Mehler, MD[c]

KEYWORDS

- Binge eating disorder • BED • Obesity • Metabolic syndrome

KEY POINTS

- Binge eating disorder is a highly prevalent and significant eating disorder with serious impairments to function and quality of life.
- Binge eating disorder is associated with many diseases associated with obesity and may confer additional medical risks to individuals with comorbidities.
- Recognition and treatment of binge eating disorder entail understanding and addressing medical comorbidities while addressing issues specific to binge eating disorder.

Binge eating disorder (BED) is the most common eating disorder with a prevalence of up to 3.5% and is more common than anorexia nervosa and bulimia nervosa combined.[1] It is defined by episodes of eating more food than most people would eat in a similar period under similar circumstances with a feeling of loss of control. Binge episodes include eating more rapidly than normal, eating until uncomfortably full, and eating large amounts of food when not hungry. Persons with BED may eat alone because of embarrassment, express feelings of disgust with one's self, and feel depressed or guilty after overeating with notable distress about binge eating. By definition, binge episodes occur at least once a week for 3 months. In BED, individuals do not regularly use compensatory behaviors like purging, fasting, or exercise.[2] BED is highly comorbid with other psychiatric disorders, including addiction, history of trauma, and adverse childhood events (ACEs).[3,4] In addition, BED is associated with significant medical morbidity, the focus of this article.[5]

OBESITY, METABOLIC SYNDROME, DIABETES, AND BARIATRIC SURGERY

Obesity is considered one of the most pressing modern public health concerns because of the cost of medical care associated with it and the costs to society through

Disclosure Statement: None of the authors have any disclosures to declare.
[a] Eating Recovery Center, 98 Spruce Street, Denver, CO 80230, USA; [b] Binge Eating Treatment and Recovery, Eating Recovery Center, Northwestern University Medical School, Department of Psychiatry, Eating Recovery Center Insight, 333 North Michigan Avenue, 19th Floor, Chicago, IL 60601, USA; [c] Eating Recovery Center, ACUTE @ Denver Health, Glassman Professor of Medicine, University of Colorado School of Medicine, 7351 East Lowry Boulevard, Suite 200, Denver, CO 80230, USA
* Corresponding author.
E-mail address: Elizabeth.Wassenaar@eatingrecovery.com

Psychiatr Clin N Am 42 (2019) 275–286
https://doi.org/10.1016/j.psc.2019.01.010
0193-953X/19/© 2019 Elsevier Inc. All rights reserved.

psych.theclinics.com

loss of productivity and impairments in the quality of life of persons affected.[6] BED is highly associated with obesity and obesity-related diseases. In a group of adults with BED, 71% had a body mass index (BMI) >30 and more than 25% of children and adolescents with obesity and overweight endorsed binge and loss of control eating.[7,8] In the Framingham Heart Study, 13.9% of those who endorsed binge eating behaviors were overweight or obese.[9] Compared with individuals with obesity without binge eating behaviors, individuals with obesity and binge eating had higher BMIs and were more impaired by psychiatric comorbidities.[10]

Metabolic syndrome is a collection of factors that are associated with an increased risk for obesity, type 2 diabetes (T2D), and cardiovascular disease.[11] Persons with BED have metabolic and inflammatory markers linked to metabolic syndrome and increased morbidity and mortality. Compared with non-BED obese matched controls, central adiposity, elevated fasting insulin levels, insulin resistance coupled with high HgA_{1c} levels, and hypertension occur more frequently in populations with BED. BED increases the risk for the development of T2D up to 13 times, and up to 25% of patients with T2D may have BED.[12,13] The cardiovascular stress response is impaired in patients with BED with less heart rate variability noted during stressful tasks, which has been shown to be an independent risk factor for morbidity.[14] Inflammatory markers, such as erythrocyte sedimentation rate, high-sensitive C-reactive protein, and white blood cell count are abnormally elevated in persons with BED and obesity versus controls.[15] Among the 30% of patients with BED without obesity, there are lower rates of the signs of metabolic disease; however, this may be related to the duration of effects of BED, because these patients tend to be younger.[8,16]

Type 1 diabetes (T1D) and other autoimmune disorders are also more common in patients with BED.[17] In persons with T1D, disinhibited eating and misuse of insulin are described in relation to disordered eating behaviors (DEB), although the coincident diagnosis of BED and T1D has rarely been identified in the literature. Binge eating episodes related to dietary restraint or hypoglycemic states can lead to disinhibited eating and are accompanied by guilt and shame about eating. The compensatory misuse of insulin is described in up to 27% of individuals for weight control with DEB, but there are minimal data on uncompensated binge episodes, an area much in need of further attention because current estimates of coincident obesity and T1D are as high as 50%.[18–22]

Nonalcoholic fatty liver disease (NAFLD) is the most common liver disease in the United States and is associated with risks for steatosis, steatohepatitis, and cirrhosis. Risk factors for NAFLD, including obesity, insulin resistance, and metabolic syndrome, are more common in patients with BED. In a pilot study, a population with NAFLD screened positive for BED in 23% of cases.[23]

Individuals with BED are overrepresented in populations seeking weight loss treatment. In bariatric surgery candidates, BED is the second most commonly diagnosed psychiatric disorder exceeded only by major depressive disorder. In preoperative samples, 4% to 49% of bariatric surgery candidates met full criteria for BED, whereas 66% reported at least one binge episode per week.[24] Prevalence rates of BED before bariatric surgery vary widely.[25] Weight reduction is associated with the lessening or resolution of comorbidities and obesity-associated mortality[26]; however, dieting and surgical weight management can be problematic in BED.[27] Dieting is associated with the onset of binge eating symptoms in both adolescents and overweight and obese adults, and calorie restriction in adults with BED may not be sustainable.[28–30] Identifying the behaviors of BED in patients seeking bariatric surgery is absolutely essential, particularly because the incidence of bariatric surgery increases. In 2017, approximately 228,000 bariatric procedures were performed in the United States, a

144% increase from 2011.[31] BED can impact the success of bariatric surgery and is associated with poorer surgical outcomes, less weight loss, more weight regain, and surgical revision.[25,32] Binge eating behaviors after bariatric surgery can result in stretching of the surgical pouch, and bariatric BED describes a binge as an amount of food that is contraindicated postsurgically based on size, content, or physical capacity.[33] Binge episodes have been described in between 6% and 64% of the post-bariatric surgery population, and more than 50% of bariatric revisions at one center were due to insufficient weight loss or weight regain.[25,34]

Other maladaptive eating behaviors can occur in patients with bariatric surgery, including plugging, dumping, and postsurgical eating avoidance disorder (PSEAD). Plugging refers to eating foods that cannot pass successfully from the surgical pouch, resulting in vomiting, whereas dumping refers to osmotic overload from calorie-dense intake resulting in fluid sequestration, nausea, diarrhea, and fatigue. PSEAD is food avoidance for reasons of weight control and can result in malnutrition.[35] Episodic vomiting occurs in up to 60% of individuals in the first 6 months after bariatric surgery, and as many as 76% of patients experience plugging within 2 years after bariatric surgery. Dumping syndrome occurs in approximately 70% of patients following gastric bypass.[36,37] The consequences of frequent vomiting or plugging may mimic health consequences of intentional purging, and conversely, intentional plugging or vomiting has also been described as a weight management strategy. Misuse of laxatives after bariatric surgery has also been described.[38,39]

"Addiction transfer" and "symptom substitution" are informal terms that have been used to describe the replacement of other compulsive and maladaptive behaviors in lieu of the maladaptive use of food following bariatric surgery. These behaviors can include alcohol or drug use, gambling, sexual behaviors, and nonsuicidal self-injury. In a large observational study of post Roux-en-Y gastric bypass patients, up to 40% of patients developed new alcohol use disorders.[40,41] Particularly in relation to the excessive use of alcohol, the additive risks of vitamin deficiencies may be significant after bariatric surgery. Therefore, it is prudent to be vigilant for the consequences of misuse of substances, self-harm, and other risky behaviors following surgery.

GASTROINTESTINAL

Gastrointestinal (GI) concerns are common in obesity and more so in patients with BED. Patients with BED report more acid reflux, dysphagia, bloating, abdominal pain, lower GI urgency, diarrhea, and constipation.[42] Dysmotility has been well described in anorexia nervosa and has also recently been described in a population with rapid weight gain (>3 kg in 3 months); however, post hoc analysis revealed an increased risk of deliberate purging after binge eating in this sample, which confounds the results.[43,44] Autoimmune gastroenterologic disorders, especially Crohn disease, may also be more prevalent in BED.[17]

In obesity research, there is an increasing interest in the gut microbiome and inflammation, psychiatric illness, and weight management. To date, there are no data examining microbiota differences in persons with BED; however, this emerging field may have much to offer to the understanding of the neurobiological aspect of BED.[45,46]

NUTRITIONAL CONCERNS

Although obesity is associated with overconsumption of calories, persons with obesity and BED are at risk for nutritional deficiencies. Analyses of the nutritional composition of binges show calorie-dense foods higher in carbohydrates and sugar, with high fat content, and lower in protein.[47–49] Higher-fat diets are associated with decreased intake of vitamins A, C, and folate, and consumption of sweetened beverages is associated with decreased intake of milk, impacting levels of calcium and vitamin D3. In individuals with more body fat, vitamin D3 may be sequestered in adipose tissue. In addition, physical limitations potentially leading to less time in the sun coupled with more skin coverage may further reduce vitamin D levels. Vitamin D and calcium deficiencies can result in decreased bone mass, and low vitamin D may have a bidirectional relationship with obesity and depression.[50–53]

Bariatric surgery may exacerbate preexisting nutritional deficiencies and/or produce new ones depending on procedure and postsurgical eating behaviors. Postsurgical adherence to vitamin and supplement recommendations is crucial to prevent deficiencies in micronutrients. This risk is increased when there is postoperative vomiting or restriction. In addition, overall functional impairments in BED and/or concurrent psychiatric illness may lead to difficulty with treatment compliance with prescribed meal plans and supplements.[50]

Protein malabsorption, common after bariatric surgery and potentially worsened by binge food choices, coupled with hypoalbuminemia can lead to hair loss and poor wound healing. Iron deficiency is common after bariatric surgery, occurring in up to 47% of patients and exacerbated by inflammatory conditions and menstruation in women. Vitamins B1 and B12 have not been evaluated in patients with BED but are impacted by obesity and bariatric surgery. Vitamin B1 deficiency is especially vulnerable to excessive postoperative vomiting or PSEAD. Zinc deficiency has been noted in up to 28% of patients with obesity presenting for bariatric surgery and increases to 51% following bariatric procedures.[54] Zinc deficiency has been identified as a target for treatment in anorexia nervosa because of its role in regulating taste and appetite, and the role of zinc in insulin resistance in obesity and BED is an area of active investigation.[55,56]

CANCER

There are multiple risk factors for cancer in persons with BED. Obesity is associated with increased morbidity and mortality from many types of cancer, including colorectal cancers, esophageal adenocarcinoma, cancers of the gallbladder, pancreas, liver, kidney, postmenopausal breast, endometrium, thyroid, ovarian and prostate, and non-Hodgkin lymphoma and multiple myeloma. T2D may further increase the risk for multiple types of cancer and mortality. In addition to obesity and T2D, the use of tobacco is associated with an increased risk of pancreatic cancer. Individuals with BED are likely to have more difficulty with smoking cessation, have more weight gain following smoking cessation, and are more likely to smoke during pregnancy.[57,58] Hypercholesterolemia and certain fatty acids that are associated with NAFLD have been found to also promote colon neoplasia in intestinal cancer.[59] Although no specific studies examining cancer rates in individuals with BED have been completed, increased risk for cancers correlating with BED could be hypothesized.[60]

REPRODUCTIVE HEALTH

Multiple morbidities related to reproductive health are associated with BED. Urinary incontinence is 3 times more likely in bariatric surgery candidates with BED and mental illness and likely impacted by consequences of both obesity and psychiatric impairment.[61,62] Menstrual concerns, such as amenorrhea, oligomenorrhea, and premenstrual dysphoric disorder, are associated with binge eating. Early menarche has not been described with BED; however, earlier menarche is described in female adolescent patients with ACES and obesity, which are associated with BED.[63–67]

Polycystic ovarian syndrome (PCOS) is correlated with insulin resistance and an increased risk of infertility. Of women with PCOS, 30% to 50% are obese or overweight, 17% to 23% of women with PCOS meet criteria for BED, and the risk of PCOS is increased by 25% in patients with BED.[61,68–70] The primary treatment of PCOS is weight management, including bariatric surgery.[71] As mentioned above, an increase in risky sexual behaviors may follow bariatric surgery in patients with BED.[41] For persons of reproductive age, discussions of safe sexual practices and contraception should be included in managing patients with BED following bariatric surgery.

In women seeking fertility treatment, BED is more common among infertile women than fertile controls. Furthermore, women with BED have an increased risk of miscarriage.[72,73] The association of infertility and BED in male patients has been mostly unexamined in the literature; however, male subfertility is associated with obesity and metabolic syndrome.[74]

Pregnancy confers some degree of protection from eating-disordered behaviors in anorexia nervosa and bulimia nervosa; however, pregnancy increases vulnerability to BED.[75] BED during pregnancy is associated with a risk for excessive gestational weight gain and an increased risk of the use of tobacco.[58,76] During pregnancy, women with BED have lower intake of folate, potassium, and vitamin C as well as a higher intake of caffeine. Excessive caffeine intake may mediate an association with spontaneous miscarriage, whereas low folate is associated with birth defects.[77] BED is associated with maternal hypertension, a prolonged duration of first and second stages of labor, and a higher rate of cesarean section and large-for-gestational-age infants. In addition, pregestational T2D and obesity increase the risk for perinatal death and birth defects.[58,78,79] In pregnant women with epilepsy, BED is more common, and there is an increased risk for preeclampsia and cesarean section. These risks may possibly be related to treatment with antiepileptic drugs (AEDs). Some AEDs are used in the treatment of binge eating and should be included in a discussion of risks for pregnancy and treatment of BED.[80,81] Last, women with BED are at increased risk of postpartum depression.[82]

Individuals with BED indicate more impairments in sexual life independent of obesity. Using the assessment of Female Sexual Function Index, a measure of satisfying sexual encounters for women, functional sexual impairment was found in individuals with BED. Sexual dysfunction was associated with dissociative episodes during sexual activity, possibly owing to the high incidence of sexual trauma in patients who manifest binge eating behaviors.[3,83–85]

NEUROLOGIC

Idiopathic intracranial hypertension, a common cause of severe headaches in obesity, is associated with BED.[86] As previously described, epilepsy and BED can cooccur during pregnancy.[80] Concerning dementias, there have been case reports of abnormal binge eating behaviors as a part of frontotemporal dementia but not Parkinson disease. The long-term risk of neurodegenerative disorders and BED has yet to be examined.[87–89]

SLEEP

There are multiple sleep abnormalities to be aware of in persons with BED. Disrupted sleep is seen more commonly in BED compared with obese controls, as demonstrated by rest-activity circadian rhythm, a measure of sleep activity.[90] In patients seeking bariatric surgery, 52% had obstructive sleep apnea, and in those patients, BED was significantly more common.[91] Night eating syndrome (NES), under Other Specified

Feeding or Eating Disorders in *Diagnostic and Statistical Manual of Mental Disorders*, Fifth Edition, is a pattern of consuming most calories following the evening meal and is associated with dysphoria, insomnia, and morning anorexia.[2] It is associated with disordered neuroendocrine function and circadian pattern abnormalities. Approximately 15% to 20% of patients with BED also have NES. NES is strongly associated with obesity, in persons seeking weight loss surgery, and with an increased risk for metabolic syndrome.[92] Narcolepsy has previously been associated with excess body weight, particularly with central adiposity, and nearly a quarter of patients with narcolepsy met criteria for disordered binge eating in one study.[93,94] Patients with BED should be screened for sleep disorders and referred for sleep studies if appropriate.

MUSCULOSKELETAL

Bone disease can be a long-term sequela of eating disorders, particularly in patients with anorexia nervosa.[95] BED is also associated with bone pathologic condition. Obesity, higher body fat percentage, and elevated cortisol levels are associated with lower bone mineral density and bone mineral content; however, the long-term outcomes of these findings are, as of yet, unknown.[96–98] Mobility concerns have been independently associated with obesity and BED in bariatric surgery candidates.[61] Obesity is a risk factor for osteoarthritis (OA) due to mechanical stress and impaired lipid metabolism, inflammation, and adipokines, such as leptin. Although the incidence of OA has not been specifically examined in the BED population, there are coincident risk factors associated with OA and BED, and an intersection could be hypothesized.[99] Furthermore, patients with fibromyalgia and obesity had more binge days than patients without obesity, and in men, binge eating was associated with significantly more neck, shoulder, and back pain and chronic muscular pain independent of BMI.[100,101]

TREATMENT CONSIDERATIONS

Treatment of BED encompasses psychological, behavioral, and medical treatment. Meta-analyses examining the efficacy of behavioral treatments have established effectiveness of cognitive behavioral therapy (CBT) and interpersonal behavioral therapy to reduce frequency of binge eating behaviors, decreasing eating disorder–related cognitions and increasing the likelihood of abstinence of binge eating behaviors.[102–104] In reviews of treatment interventions, therapist-led CBT showed superiority to wait-list or self-help control groups.[105]

Treatment opportunities for patients with BED are limited by poor recognition of the disorder by both individuals and health care professionals. Patients with BED may be referred for treatment of medical comorbidities without specialized eating disorder treatment that can address the disorder at multiple levels. Guidelines for higher levels of care in eating disorder treatment have been skewed toward patients who are significantly below ideal body weight or are experiencing medical consequences of purging. Higher levels of care for patients with BED can address psychiatric, medical, and/or nutritional instability, and containment may be necessary to interrupt "automatic," impulsive, and/or compulsive binge eating behaviors.

SUMMARY

In summary, like other eating disorders, BED presents with medical comorbidity in almost every system in the body and can have devastating consequences on quality and length of life. It is the most common eating disorder and yet has been underidentified and mismanaged in medical settings.[106] Individuals with obesity-related diseases are vulnerable to internalized stigma and may avoid necessary health care for fear of stigmatized assessments.[107,108] Improved understanding of the presentation and pathologic condition of BED and interrelated conditions will allow us to continue to make meaningful progress in providing care for these individuals, who are at major risk for morbidity and mortality.

REFERENCES

1. Hudson JI, Hiripi E, Pope HG, et al. The prevalence and correlates of eating disorders in the national comorbidity survey replication. Biol Psychiatry 2007;61(3): 348–58.
2. American Psychiatric Association. Diagnostic and statistical manual of mental disorders. 5th edition. Washington, DC: American Psychiatric Publishing; 2013.
3. Palmisano GL, Innamorati M, Vanderlinden J. Life adverse experiences in relation with obesity and binge eating disorder: a systematic review. J Behav Addict 2016;5(1):11–31.
4. Kessler RC, Berglund PA, Chiu WT, et al. The prevalence and correlates of binge eating disorder in the World Health Organization World Mental Health Surveys. Biol Psychiatry 2013;73(9):904–14.
5. Olguin P, Fuentes M, Gabler G, et al. Medical comorbidity of binge eating disorder. Eat Weight Disord 2017;22(1):13–26.
6. U.S. Department of Health & Human Services. Adult obesity causes & consequences | Overweight & obesity | CDC 2018. Available at: https://www.cdc.gov/obesity/adult/causes.html. Accessed October 25, 2018.
7. He J, Cai Z, Fan X. Prevalence of binge and loss of control eating among children and adolescents with overweight and obesity: an exploratory meta-analysis. Int J Eat Disord 2017;50(2):91–103.
8. Dingemans AE, van Furth EF. Binge Eating Disorder psychopathology in normal weight and obese individuals. Int J Eat Disord 2012;45(1):135–8.
9. Abraham TM, Massaro JM, Hoffmann U, et al. Metabolic characterization of adults with binge eating in the general population: the framingham heart study. Obesity (Silver Spring) 2014;22(11):2441–9.
10. da Luz FQ, Hay P, Touyz S, et al. Obesity with comorbid eating disorders: associated health risks and treatment approaches. Nutrients 2018;10(7). https://doi.org/10.3390/nu10070829.
11. Rosenzweig JL, Ferrannini E, Grundy SM, et al. Primary prevention of cardiovascular disease and type 2 diabetes in patients at metabolic risk: an endocrine society clinical practice guideline. J Clin Endocrinol Metab 2008; 93(10):3671–89.
12. Raevuori A, Suokas J, Haukka J, et al. Highly increased risk of type 2 diabetes in patients with binge eating disorder and bulimia nervosa. Int J Eat Disord 2015; 48(6):555–62.
13. Hudson JI, Lalonde JK, Coit CE, et al. Longitudinal study of the diagnosis of components of the metabolic syndrome in individuals with binge-eating disorder. Am J Clin Nutr 2010;91(6):1568–73.
14. Messerli-Bürgy N, Engesser C, Lemmenmeier E, et al. Cardiovascular stress reactivity and recovery in bulimia nervosa and binge eating disorder. Int J Psychophysiol 2010;78(2):163–8.

15. Succurro E, Segura-Garcia C, Ruffo M, et al. Obese patients with a binge eating disorder have an unfavorable metabolic and inflammatory profile. Medicine (Baltimore) 2015;94(52):e2098.
16. Thornton LM, Watson HJ, Jangmo A, et al. Binge-eating disorder in the Swedish national registers: somatic comorbidity. Int J Eat Disord 2017;50(1):58–65.
17. Raevuori A, Haukka J, Vaarala O, et al. The increased risk for autoimmune diseases in patients with eating disorders. PLoS One 2014;9(8):e104845.
18. Colton PA, Olmsted MP, Daneman D, et al. Eating disorders in girls and women with type 1 diabetes: a longitudinal study of prevalence, onset, remission, and recurrence. Diabetes Care 2015;38(7):1212–7.
19. Peterson CM, Fischer S, Young-Hyman D. Topical review: a comprehensive risk model for disordered eating in youth with type 1 diabetes. J Pediatr Psychol 2015;40(4):385–90.
20. Merwin RM, Moskovich AA, Dmitrieva NO, et al. Disinhibited eating and weight-related insulin mismanagement among individuals with type 1 diabetes. Appetite 2014;81:123–30.
21. Mottalib A, Kasetty M, Mar JY, et al. Weight management in patients with type 1 diabetes and obesity. Curr Diab Rep 2017;17(10). https://doi.org/10.1007/s11892-017-0918-8.
22. Takii M, Uchigata Y, Nozaki T, et al. Classification of type 1 diabetic females with bulimia nervosa into subgroups according to purging behavior. Diabetes Care 2002;25(9):1571–5.
23. Zhang J. Pilot study of the prevalence of binge eating disorder in non-alcoholic fatty liver disease patients. Ann Gastroenterol 2017. https://doi.org/10.20524/aog.2017.0200.
24. Williams GA, Hawkins MAW, Duncan J, et al. Maladaptive eating behavior assessment among bariatric surgery candidates: evaluation of the Eating Disorder Diagnostic Scale. Surg Obes Relat Dis 2017;13(7):1183–8.
25. Conceição EM, Utzinger LM, Pisetsky EM. Eating disorders and problematic eating behaviours before and after bariatric surgery: characterization, assessment and association with treatment outcomes. Eur Eat Disord Rev 2015; 23(6):417–25.
26. Wolfe BM, Kvach E, Eckel RH. Treatment of obesity: weight loss and bariatric surgery. Circ Res 2016;118(11):1844–55.
27. Meyer LB, Waaddegaard M, Lau ME, et al. (Dis-)solving the weight problem in binge-eating disorder: systemic insights from three treatment contexts with weight stability, weight loss, and weight acceptance. Qual Health Res 2018. https://doi.org/10.1177/1049732318764874. 1049732318764874.
28. Goldschmidt AB, Wall M, Loth KA, et al. Which dieters are at risk for the onset of binge-eating? A prospective study of adolescents and young adults. J Adolesc Health 2012;51(1):86–92.
29. da Luz FQ, Hay P, Gibson AA, et al. Does severe dietary energy restriction increase binge eating in overweight or obese individuals? A systematic review. Obes Rev 2015;16(8):652–65.
30. Wonderlich SA, de Zwaan M, Mitchell JE, et al. Psychological and dietary treatments of binge eating disorder: Conceptual implications. Int J Eat Disord 2003; 34(S1):S58–73.
31. Estimate of bariatric surgery numbers, 2011-2017. American society for metabolic and bariatric surgery. Available at: https://asmbs.org/resources/estimate-of-bariatric-surgery-numbers. Accessed October 25, 2018.

32. Brethauer SA, Kothari S, Sudan R, et al. Systematic review on reoperative bariatric surgery. Surg Obes Relat Dis 2014;10(5):952–72.
33. Ivezaj V, Barnes RD, Cooper Z, et al. Loss-of-control eating after bariatric/sleeve gastrectomy surgery: similar to binge-eating disorder despite differences in quantities. Gen Hosp Psychiatry 2018;54:25–30.
34. Park JY, Song D, Kim YJ. Causes and outcomes of revisional bariatric surgery: initial experience at a single center. Ann Surg Treat Res 2014;86(6):295–301.
35. Segal A, Kinoshita Kussunoki D, Aparecida Larino M. Post-surgical refusal to eat: anorexia nervosa, bulimia nervosa or a new eating disorder? a case series. Obes Surg 2004;14(3):353–60.
36. Still C, Sarwer DB, Blankenship J. The ASMBS textbook of bariatric surgery, vol. 2. New York: Integrated Health; Springer; 2014.
37. Ziegler O, Sirveaux MA, Brunaud L, et al. Medical follow up after bariatric surgery: nutritional and drug issues General recommendations for the prevention and treatment of nutritional deficiencies. Diabetes Metab 2009;35(6): 544–57.
38. Conceição E, Orcutt M, Mitchell J, et al. Characterization of eating disorders after bariatric surgery: a case series study. Int J Eat Disord 2013;46(3):274–9.
39. de Zwaan M, Hilbert A, Swan-Kremeier L, et al. Comprehensive interview assessment of eating behavior 18-35 months after gastric bypass surgery for morbid obesity. Surg Obes Relat Dis 2010;6(1):79–85.
40. Tækker L, Christensen BJ, Lunn S. From bingeing to cutting: the substitution of a mal-adaptive coping strategy after bariatric surgery. J Eat Disord 2018;6:24.
41. Mitchell JE, Steffen K, Engel S, et al. Addictive disorders after Roux-en-Y gastric bypass. Surg Obes Relat Dis 2015;11(4):897–905.
42. Cremonini F, Camilleri M, Clark MM, et al. Associations among binge eating behavior patterns and gastrointestinal symptoms: a population-based study. Int J Obes 2009;33(3):342–53.
43. Eslick GD, Howell SC, Talley NJ. Dysmotility symptoms are independently associated with weight change: a population-based study of australian adults. J Neurogastroenterol Motil 2015;21(4):603–11.
44. Benini L, Todesco T, Dalle Grave R, et al. Gastric emptying in patients with restricting and binge/purging subtypes of anorexia nervosa. Am J Gastroenterol 2004;99(8):1448–54.
45. Mangiola F, Ianiro G, Franceschi F, et al. Gut microbiota in autism and mood disorders. World J Gastroenterol 2016;22(1):361–8.
46. Castaner O, Goday A, Park Y-M, et al. The gut microbiome profile in obesity: a systematic review. Int J Endocrinol 2018;2018:4095789.
47. Gayle JL, Fitzgibbon ML, Martinovich Z. A preliminary analysis of binge episodes: comparison of a treatment-seeking sample of Black and White women. Eat Behav 2004;5(4):303–13.
48. Horvath JDC, Kops NL, de Castro MLD, et al. Food consumption in patients referred for bariatric surgery with and without binge eating disorder. Eat Behav 2015;19:173–6.
49. Agras WS, Telch CF. The effects of caloric deprivation and negative affect on binge eating in obese binge-eating disordered women. Behav Ther 1998; 29(3):491–503.
50. Pawaskar M, Witt EA, Supina D, et al. Impact of binge eating disorder on functional impairment and work productivity in an adult community sample in the United States. Int J Clin Pract 2017;71(7). https://doi.org/10.1111/ijcp.12970.

51. Dix CF, Bauer JD, Martin I, et al. Association of sun exposure, skin colour and body mass index with Vitamin D status in individuals who are morbidly obese. Nutrients 2017;9(10). https://doi.org/10.3390/nu9101094.

52. Compston JE, Vedi S, Ledger JE, et al. Vitamin D status and bone histomorphometry in gross obesity. Am J Clin Nutr 1981;34(11):2359–63.

53. Cizza G. Major depressive disorder is a risk factor for low bone mass, central obesity, and other medical conditions. Dialogues Clin Neurosci 2011;13(1): 73–87.

54. Xanthakos SA. Nutritional deficiencies in obesity and after bariatric surgery. Pediatr Clin North Am 2009;56(5):1105–21.

55. Cruz KJC, Morais JBS, de Oliveira ARS, et al. The Effect of zinc supplementation on insulin resistance in obese subjects: a systematic review. Biol Trace Elem Res 2017;176(2):239–43.

56. Barron LJ, Barron RF, Johnson JCS, et al. A retrospective analysis of biochemical and haematological parameters in patients with eating disorders. J Eat Disord 2017;5:32.

57. Chao A, White MA, Grilo CM. Smoking status and psychosocial factors in binge eating disorder and bulimia nervosa. Eat Behav 2016;21:54–8.

58. Bulik CM, Von Holle A, Siega-Riz AM, et al. Birth outcomes in women with eating disorders in the norwegian mother and child cohort study (MoBa). Int J Eat Disord 2009;42(1):9–18.

59. Berger NA. Obesity and cancer pathogenesis. Ann N Y Acad Sci 2014;1311: 57–76.

60. Brewster DH, Nowell SL, Clark DN. Risk of oesophageal cancer among patients previously hospitalised with eating disorder. Cancer Epidemiol 2015;39(3): 313–20.

61. Mitchell JE, King WC, Pories W, et al. Binge eating disorder and medical comorbidities in bariatric surgery candidates. Int J Eat Disord 2015;48(5):471–6.

62. Subak LL, Richter HE, Hunskaar S. Obesity and urinary incontinence: epidemiology and clinical research update. J Urol 2009;182(6 Suppl):S2–7.

63. Algars M, Huang L, Von Holle AF, et al. Binge eating and menstrual dysfunction. J Psychosom Res 2014;76(1):19–22.

64. Bell JA, Carslake D, Wade KH, et al. Influence of puberty timing on adiposity and cardiometabolic traits: a Mendelian randomisation study. PLoS Med 2018; 15(8). https://doi.org/10.1371/journal.pmed.1002641.

65. Hartman S, Li Z, Nettle D, et al. External-environmental and internal-health early life predictors of adolescent development. Dev Psychopathol 2017;29(5): 1839–49.

66. Liu Y, Sun Y, Tao F, et al. Associations between adverse childhood experiences with early puberty timing and possible gender difference. Zhonghua Liu Xing Bing Xue Za Zhi 2015;36(4):314–7 [in Chinese].

67. Dahlgren CL, Qvigstad E. Eating disorders in premenstrual dysphoric disorder: a neuroendocrinological pathway to the pathogenesis and treatment of binge eating. J Eat Disord 2018;6. https://doi.org/10.1186/s40337-018-0222-2.

68. Kerchner A, Lester W, Stuart SP, et al. Risk of depression and other mental health disorders in women with polycystic ovary syndrome: a longitudinal study. Fertil Steril 2009;91(1):207–12.

69. Lee I, Cooney LG, Saini S, et al. Increased risk of disordered eating in polycystic ovary syndrome. Fertil Steril 2017;107(3):796–802.

70. Zain MM, Norman RJ. Impact of obesity on female fertility and fertility treatment. Womens Health 2008;4(2):183–94.

71. Sirmans S, Pate K. Epidemiology, diagnosis, and management of polycystic ovary syndrome. Clin Epidemiol 2013;1. https://doi.org/10.2147/CLEP.S37559.
72. Linna MS, Raevuori A, Haukka J, et al. Reproductive health outcomes in eating disorders. Int J Eat Disord 2013;46(8):826–33.
73. Kimmel MC, Ferguson EH, Zerwas S, et al. Obstetric and gynecologic problems associated with eating disorders. Int J Eat Disord 2016;49(3):260–75.
74. McPherson NO, Lane M. Male obesity and subfertility, is it really about increased adiposity? Asian J Androl 2015;17(3):450–8.
75. Bulik CM, Von Holle A, Hamer R, et al. Patterns of remission, continuation, and incidence of broadly defined eating disorders during early pregnancy in the Norwegian Mother and Child Cohort Study (MoBa). Psychol Med 2007;37(8): 1109–18.
76. Siega-Riz AM, Von Holle A, Haugen M, et al. Gestational weight gain of women with eating disorders in the Norwegian pregnancy cohort. Int J Eat Disord 2011; 44(5):428–34.
77. Siega-Riz AM, Haugen M, Meltzer HM, et al. Nutrient and food group intakes of women with and without Bulimia Nervosa and Binge Eating Disorder during pregnancy. Am J Clin Nutr 2008;87(5):1346–55.
78. Linna MS, Raevuori A, Haukka J, et al. Pregnancy, obstetric, and perinatal health outcomes in eating disorders. Am J Obstet Gynecol 2014;211(4):392.e1-8.
79. Mitanchez D, Yzydorczyk C, Simeoni U. What neonatal complications should the pediatrician be aware of in case of maternal gestational diabetes? World J Diabetes 2015;6(5):734–43.
80. Kolstad E, Gilhus NE, Veiby G, et al. Epilepsy and eating disorders during pregnancy: Prevalence, complications and birth outcome. Seizure 2015;28:81–4.
81. TOXNET. Available at: https://toxnet.nlm.nih.gov/cgi-bin/sis/search2. Accessed November 8, 2018.
82. Mazzeo SE, Slof-Op't Landt MCT, Jones I, et al. Associations among postpartum depression, eating disorders, and perfectionism in a population-based sample of adult women. Int J Eat Disord 2006;39(3):202–11.
83. Castellini G, Mannucci E, Mazzei C, et al. Sexual function in obese women with and without binge eating disorder. J Sex Med 2010;7(12):3969–78.
84. Castellini G, Lo Sauro C, Ricca V, et al. Body esteem as a common factor of a tendency toward binge eating and sexual dissatisfaction among women: the role of dissociation and stress response during sex. J Sex Med 2017;14(8):1036–45.
85. Rieger E, Wilfley DE, Stein RI, et al. A comparison of quality of life in obese individuals with and without binge eating disorder. Int J Eat Disord 2005;37(3):234–40.
86. Raggi A, Curone M, Bianchi Marzoli S, et al. Impact of obesity and binge eating disorder on patients with idiopathic intracranial hypertension. Cephalalgia 2017; 37(3):278–83.
87. Singam C, Walterfang M, Mocellin R, et al. Topiramate for abnormal eating behaviour in frontotemporal dementia. Behav Neurol 2013;27(3):285–6.
88. Shinagawa S, Tsuno N, Nakayama K. Managing abnormal eating behaviours in frontotemporal lobar degeneration patients with topiramate. Psychogeriatrics 2013;13(1):58–61.
89. Solla P, Cannas A, Floris GL, et al. Behavioral, neuropsychiatric and cognitive disorders in Parkinson's disease patients with and without motor complications. Prog Neuropsychopharmacol Biol Psychiatry 2011;35(4):1009–13.
90. Roveda E, Montaruli A, Galasso L, et al. Rest-activity circadian rhythm and sleep quality in patients with binge eating disorder. Chronobiol Int 2018; 35(2):198–207.

91. Sockalingam S, Tehrani H, Taube-Schiff M, et al. The relationship between eating psychopathology and obstructive sleep apnea in bariatric surgery candidates: a retrospective study. Int J Eat Disord 2017;50(7):801–7.

92. McCuen-Wurst C, Ruggieri M, Allison KC. Disordered eating and obesity: associations between binge-eating disorder, night-eating syndrome, and weight-related comorbidities. Ann N Y Acad Sci 2018;1411(1):96–105.

93. Morse AM, Sanjeev K. Narcolepsy and Psychiatric Disorders: Comorbidities or Shared Pathophysiology? Med Sci (Basel) 2018;6(1). https://doi.org/10.3390/medsci6010016.

94. Fortuyn HAD, Swinkels S, Buitelaar J, et al. High prevalence of eating disorders in narcolepsy with cataplexy: a case-control study. Sleep 2008;31(3):335–41.

95. Drabkin A, Rothman MS, Wassenaar E, et al. Assessment and clinical management of bone disease in adults with eating disorders: a review. J Eat Disord 2017;5. https://doi.org/10.1186/s40337-017-0172-0.

96. Schvey NA, Tanofsky-Kraff M, Yanoff LB, et al. Disordered-eating attitudes in relation to bone mineral density and markers of bone turnover in overweight adolescents. J Adolesc Health 2009;45(1):33–9.

97. Mosca LN, Goldberg TBL, da Silva VN, et al. Excess body fat negatively affects bone mass in adolescents. Nutrition 2014;30(7–8):847–52.

98. Mathisen TF, Rosenvinge JH, Friborg O, et al. Body composition and physical fitness in women with bulimia nervosa or binge-eating disorder. Int J Eat Disord 2018;51(4):331–42.

99. Thijssen E, van Caam A, van der Kraan PM. Obesity and osteoarthritis, more than just wear and tear: pivotal roles for inflamed adipose tissue and dyslipidaemia in obesity-induced osteoarthritis. Rheumatologe (Oxford) 2015;54(4):588–600.

100. Senna MK, Ahmad HS, Fathi W. Depression in obese patients with primary fibromyalgia: the mediating role of poor sleep and eating disorder features. Clin Rheumatol 2013;32(3):369–75.

101. Reichborn-Kjennerud T, Bulik CM, Sullivan PF, et al. Psychiatric and medical symptoms in binge eating in the absence of compensatory behaviors. Obes Res 2004;12(9):1445–54.

102. Wilson GT, Wilfley DE, Agras WS, et al. Psychological treatments of binge eating disorder. Arch Gen Psychiatry 2010;67(1):94.

103. Wilfley DE, Welch RR, Stein RI, et al. A randomized comparison of group cognitive-behavioral therapy and group interpersonal psychotherapy for the treatment of overweight individuals with binge-eating disorder. Arch Gen Psychiatry 2002;59(8):713.

104. Brownley KA, Berkman ND, Peat CM, et al. Binge-eating disorder in adults: a systematic review and meta-analysis. Ann Intern Med 2016;165(6):409.

105. Ghaderi A, Odeberg J, Gustafsson S, et al. Psychological, pharmacological, and combined treatments for binge eating disorder: a systematic review and meta-analysis. Peer J 2018;6:e5113.

106. Herman BK, Safikhani S, Hengerer D, et al. The patient experience with DSM-5-defined binge eating disorder: characteristics, barriers to treatment, and implications for primary care physicians. Postgrad Med 2014;126(5):52–63.

107. Flint SW, Oliver EJ, Copeland RJ. Editorial: obesity stigma in healthcare: impacts on policy, practice, and patients. Front Psychol 2017;8:2149.

108. Ashmore JA, Friedman KE, Reichmann SK, et al. Weight-based stigmatization, psychological distress, & binge eating behavior among obese treatment-seeking adults. Eat Behav 2008;9(2):203–9.

Special Topics

Problematic Eating Behaviors and Eating Disorders Associated with Bariatric Surgery

Cassie S. Brode, PhD[a],*, James E. Mitchell, MD[b,1]

KEYWORDS

- Obesity • Bariatric surgery • Weight loss surgery • Eating disorders
- Problematic eating behaviors • Binge eating • Loss-of-control eating

KEY POINTS

- Obesity prevalence has reached epidemic proportions worldwide, and obesity results in a variety of potentially life-threatening illnesses.
- Bariatric surgery is the only effective treatment of severe obesity.
- Bariatric surgery candidates often report problematic eating symptoms.
- Loss-of-control eating and other problematic eating behaviors after bariatric surgery are associated with attenuated long-term weight loss and need to be identified and addressed.

INTRODUCTION

Obesity is increasing in prevalence worldwide and is frequently characterized as an epidemic.[1] Obesity is associated with several serious potentially life-threatening medical comorbidities, including type 2 diabetes mellitus, hypertension, dyslipidemia, sleep apnea, and cardiovascular disease.[2–5] The most effective treatment of severe obesity, and the only intervention that usually results in both substantial weight loss and resolution of or improvement in most weight-related comorbidities, is bariatric surgery.[2] Two large, long-term prospective trials have clearly documented this. In

Disclosure Statement: The authors have no conflict of interest and no relationships or financial interests to disclose.
[a] Department of Behavioral Medicine and Psychiatry, West Virginia University School of Medicine, 930 Chestnut Ridge Road, Morgantown, WV 26505, USA; [b] Department of Psychiatry and Behavioral Science, University of North Dakota School of Medicine and Health Sciences, Grand Forks, ND, USA
[1] Present address: Working Office: 1244 Wildwood Way, Chaska, MN 55318.
* Corresponding author.
E-mail address: cassie.brode@hsc.wvu.edu

the controlled nonrandomized Swedish Obese Subjects study, bariatric surgery has been found to yield significant and sustained benefits in health status and health-related quality of life (HRQOL).[6–8] In the United States, the Longitudinal Assessment of Bariatric Surgery (LABS) study has yielded similarly promising findings at 7-year follow-up.[9]

Currently the most frequently performed bariatric surgeries are sleeve gastrectomy (SG), and Roux-en-Y gastric bypass (RYGB).[2] RYGB now accounts for the minority of bariatric surgeries performed in the United States and involves surgically partitioning the stomach to create a small gastric pouch, which is connected to the jejunum, bypassing the first part of the small intestine, the duodenum. SG involves surgically dividing the stomach vertically to reduce its size, creating a sleeve. SG is currently the most commonly performed bariatric surgery in the United States.

Traditionally, weight loss and remission of weight-related comorbidities were believed a result of the anatomic changes secondary to the surgery. A growing body of research suggests, however, that the mechanisms by which the RYGB, and likely the SG, lead to weight loss are through alterations in gastrointestinal physiology that include changes in the activity of certain gut hormones, bile acids, inflammatory factors, and gut bacteria (the microbiome).[10–14] These alterations in physiology have also been shown to be involved in bidirectional communication with the central nervous system.[10] Further understanding of the mechanisms of weight loss and disease remission will likely continue to be an important focus of research, because evidence suggests that postsurgery outcomes are dependent on these physiologic changes and the interactions among them.

EATING PROBLEMS IN INDIVIDUALS WITH OBESITY

Although obesity is not classified as an eating disorder, various eating problems, including overconsumption relative to energy expenditure, and problems with binge eating and night eating syndrome (NES), wherein people get up to eat during the night after having been asleep and/or eat excessively late in the evening after the evening meal, have been described.[15]

EATING PROBLEMS IN BARIATRIC SURGERY CANDIDATES

Bariatric surgery candidates have higher rates of eating problems and eating disorders compared with individuals in the general population[16,17] as well as with those with lesser degrees of obesity who seek nonsurgical treatments.[18] Bariatric surgery candidates also report substantial impairments in HRQOL,[19] are more focused on their weight and shape,[20,21] and report experiencing weight-related stigma from others,[22] which can exacerbate eating disorder symptoms[22] and increase weight via activation of stress-induced physiologic processes.[23] For example, consuming high-calorie foods, such as sweets and fats, can trigger physiologic responses that can contribute to binge eating, resulting in decreased distress or positive emotions.[24] Thus, it is not surprising that patients in greater distress and with disordered eating behaviors, such as binge eating, may present for bariatric surgery (rather than seeking more conservative weight loss methods) because patients want to achieve more rapid and sustainable weight loss to alleviate physical and psychosocial comorbidities.

This article reviews presurgical and postsurgical problematic and eating disordered behaviors that are common among bariatric surgery patients and includes the associations of these behaviors with HRQOL, psychopathology, and weight loss outcomes, concluding with treatment recommendations.

PRESURGERY
Binge Eating and Binge-eating Disorder

According to the *Diagnostic and Statistical Manual of Mental Disorders* (Fifth Edition) (*DSM-5*) criteria,[20] binge-eating disorder (BED) is defined as eating an unusually large amount of food in a short period of time (approximately 2 hours) and must be accompanied by a sense of loss of control (LOC) over eating (ie, feeling that one cannot stop eating or control the amount of food eaten). To meet the minimum diagnostic criteria for mild BED, a patient must engage in binge eating at least once per week for the past 3 months, and the binge eating must cause marked distress. Relevant to bariatric surgery candidates, recent studies have shown that the severity of BED is associated with the severity of obesity and psychopathology.[21] For example, higher perceived LOC over eating is related to greater distress and psychopathology,[25] with depressive and anxiety disorders among the most common psychiatric comorbidities.[26] Patients with BED are also more likely to have other problematic eating behaviors.[27]

BED is the most common eating disorder among bariatric surgery candidates. A recent LABS study[28] found that 10% of patients met full criteria for the disorder, which is a conservative estimate based on structured diagnostic assessments and the more stringent diagnostic criteria used in the *Diagnostic and Statistical Manual of Mental Disorders* (Fourth Edition). This well exceeds prevalence rates of BED in the general population (approximately 1.2%)[17] and is also high considering that bariatric surgery candidates tend to underreport and minimize symptoms so that they are not excluded from having surgery.[29] Most patients with BED seek treatment of their obesity rather than for an eating disorder or problematic eating behaviors.[21]

Rates of BED have varied considerably across studies[10,30] due to methodological differences, including over-reliance on self-report instruments and retrospective accounts versus structured clinical assessments.[31] In addition, there is currently no standardized approach to conducting the presurgical psychological interview, which can lead to biased estimates of BED and psychopathology. Ideally, clinicians and researchers evaluate current eating and other forms of psychopathology using gold standard approaches, such as the Eating Disorders Examination (EDE),[32] a structured clinical interview that assesses dietary restraint as well as eating, weight, and shape concerns and has been adapted for use with bariatric surgery patients (EDE Bariatric Surgery Version [EDE-BSV]), and the Structured Clinical Interview for *DSM-5* disorders,[33] respectively. The EDE is lengthy to administer and requires training, so it is not widely used[31] but does have a validated questionnaire form, the EDE-Q,[34] that can be used instead. Other validated eating disorder questionnaires, including the Eating Inventory,[35] can be used to assess cognitive restraint over eating, LOC eating, or disinhibited eating, and hunger.

Another area of interest in the past several years has been to determine whether presurgical binge eating or BED is related to suboptimal weight loss outcomes after bariatric surgery. Numerous studies have been conducted, but a majority do not support a relationship, and only a few support that BED is related to poorer weight loss outcomes.[31] For this reason, binge eating or BED is not considered to be a contraindication for bariatric surgery. Patients with presurgical binge eating/BED, however, should be closely monitored after surgery[31] because there is compelling evidence that disordered eating behaviors can re-emerge after surgery.[31,36–38]

Picking and Nibbling/Grazing

Picking and nibbling (P&N) is defined as unplanned and repetitive eating in-between meals and snacks, where it is unknown how much food will be eaten at the outset.[39] The term is often used interchangeably with grazing.[36,40] P&N/grazing is prevalent among patients with eating disorders,[39] including anorexia nervosa (AN), bulimia nervosa (BN), and BED, and those pursuing bariatric surgery[40] but do not seem associated with other eating disordered behaviors or psychopathology.[39] This may be because LOC eating is not included in the definition of P&N. To date, it is unclear whether or not P&N is a normative, disordered, or maladaptive eating behavior, and this is even less clear among bariatric surgery candidates, who may engage in P&N to restrict eating in an attempt to lose weight.[39] There is evidence, however, that those who engage in grazing presurgery may be more likely to continue this behavior after surgery,[36] which, as discussed later, has a deleterious effect on weight loss. Thus, these individuals may benefit from interventions that focus on eating consistent, planned meals.[41]

Night Eating Syndrome

NES is characterized by a normal sleep-wake cycle but with recurrent episodes of night eating, in which a person awakens from sleep to eat (ie, nocturnal ingestions), and by excessive food consumption (>25% of daily food intake) after the evening meal (ie, evening hyperphagia) occurring at least twice per week,[10,42] a pattern considered to be a delay in the circadian intake of food.[43] In the *DSM-5*, NES is classified as an "Other Specified Feeding or Eating Disorder,"[20] which, to be diagnosed, necessitates that individuals have

1. An awareness of their eating (which differentiates NES from a parasomnia, in which there is limited or no recollection of eating)
2. Significant distress associated with it
3. The behavior is not better explained by another disorder, such as BED

For those with NES, the amount of food eaten typically is less than what would be consumed during a binge-eating episode.[44] Approximately 15% to 20% of patients with obesity, however, do meet full criteria for both NES and BED.[36,44]

Approximately 17% of bariatric surgery candidates have NES, according to recent estimates,[27,31,44] although lower and higher rates have been reported.[30] The Night Eating Questionnaire (NEQ),[42] the most widely used, validated, self-report measure of night eating, can be used in conjunction with a diagnostic interview and a 24-hour food recall[42] to assess NES in bariatric patients.[10,27] The presence of presurgical NES, however, is not a contraindication to surgery. Rather, the NEQ can be used to monitor candidates before and after surgery and to guide interventions because NES has been associated with higher rates of lifetime anxiety, substance use, and depressive disorders[44] and is more likely to occur under periods of high stress (see de Zwaan and colleagues,[44] for a review of studies).

Associations with Psychopathology and Quality of Life

Presurgical eating disordered behaviors, in particular binge eating, have been associated with significant psychopathology, including higher rates of depression,[21] mood disorders,[26] less perceived interpersonal support, alcohol use,[27] and lower HRQOL, defined as the impact of health on an individual's functioning,[45] including, but not limited to, physical and mental health domains. These are typically significantly impaired in bariatric surgery candidates.[46,47] These impairments seem even greater among those with the highest severity of obesity as well as those with current and/ or lifetime psychiatric disorders.[18]

EATING PROBLEMS AFTER BARIATRIC SURGERY

In bariatric surgery research, weight loss has usually been used as the primary outcome, with resolution of medical comorbidities also emphasized; eating behaviors have received less attention.[31] Several recent studies show, however, that problematic eating contributes to suboptimal weight loss trajectories[48] and weight regain. A smaller percentage of patients also may develop postsurgical eating disorders, such as AN. Therefore, assessment of eating behaviors after surgery requires that clinicians understand what motivates patients to engage in these behaviors,[31] discussed later.

Loss-of-Control Eating

Although binge eating is physically not possible after bariatric surgery due to anatomic changes and consequently, improves afterward,[49] patients may still struggle with LOC eating and subjective binge-eating episodes.[49] It seems that those most at risk are patients who met criteria for BED prior to surgery.[37]

Conceição and colleagues[48] estimated that approximately 10% of patients developed LOC eating approximately 2 years after surgery, although it may re-emerge as early as 6 months postsurgery.[36,50] LOC eating is problematic because it is associated with more postsurgical complications[31,38] (eg, vomiting), higher psychopathology (eg, depression), low HRQOL,[36,37,50] eating disordered behaviors,[50] less weight loss[37] including poor long-term weight loss,[51] and greater weight regain.[52,53] It has been suggested that because patients are no longer able to engage in binge eating after surgery, prior LOC eating might present as grazing/P&N.[40] Thus, suboptimal weight loss and weight regain may result not only from disinhibited eating but also because, over time, patients are able to consume larger amounts of food.[54]

Therefore, it is critical to identify postoperative patients at risk for LOC eating and to monitor their eating behaviors and weight loss progress,[55] using the EDE-BSV,[28] for example, which more accurately assesses eating disordered behaviors after bariatric surgery. Patients identified as having LOC eating and comorbid psychopathology may then benefit from a targeted intervention that addresses both. These patients, however, may need additional support to remain engaged in treatment because there is evidence that patients with BED/LOC eating may be less adherent to postoperative dietary recommendations[54] and are less likely to attend postoperative appointments.[56]

Picking and Nibbling/Grazing

P&N/grazing is the most frequent problematic eating behavior after surgery,[49,57] affecting approximately 30% of bariatric patients.[48] Some patients develop a new onset of P&N postsurgery, although a risk factor is preoperative LOC eating.[48] The difficulty with differentiating P&N from normative eating behavior[38] is that patients are required to eat several small meals throughout the day after surgery. P&N is done, however, without planning and forethought, which often leads to the consumption of high-calorie foods or drinks.[31] In turn, P&N has been associated with postoperative weight regain,[48,49] although additional research is needed to better characterize this phenomenon and its relationship to weight outcomes.

Night Eating Syndrome

Currently, there is limited research on NES after bariatric surgery. A recent review[58] noted, however, that it occurs less frequently postsurgery. One study found a decrease in night eating from presurgery to postsurgery (from 17.1% to 7.8%) at 1-year follow-up, but this study was limited to patients having laparoscopic adjustable gastric banding.[36] Another study suggested that postoperative night eating symptoms improved among patients who had preoperative depressed mood versus those without it, but the relationship between mood and NES is complex; other factors including sleep may also play a role.[59] For example, sleep problems and depressive symptoms typically improve for most patients in the short term after surgery. Further, NES is currently defined based on the timing of eating rather than the size of eating episodes; therefore, investigators believe that patients may still engage in night eating after surgery but eat smaller amounts.[59] Therefore, future studies are needed that assess night eating prospectively across bariatric patients.[58]

Associations with Psychopathology and Quality of Life

HRQOL generally improves in the early postoperative period, particularly for physical and mental domains.[45,46,58,60] There seems, however, to be emerging evidence that these gains may be short lived,[58,61] and a subset of patients may be at risk for ongoing mood and eating problems after surgery.[27]

For example, the studies that showed improvements in mental HRQOL for long-term follow-up also noted that these gains were related to weight loss but began to decline over time.[46,61,62] Furthermore, for those with significant eating disorder symptoms after surgery, BED was associated with poor HRQOL after surgery and grazing 2 or more times per week,[52] and this was also true in another study having long-term follow-up, in which binge eating negatively affected mental HRQOL nearly 14 years after surgery.[63]

Thus, although positive changes in HRQOL and eating typically are observed in the early postoperative period,[46] there seems more variability in outcomes in the later postoperative years, which, in some studies, has been dependent on the type of surgery and related to the amount of weight lost.[45] A limitation of the literature on psychosocial outcomes after surgery is that, with the exception of a few studies,[46,63] the data have been limited to studies with outcomes at 2 years to 3 years postsurgery. Longer-term follow-up research is needed.[58]

Associations with Weight Loss Outcomes

Recent studies indicate that although problematic and disordered eating behaviors generally improve after surgery, recurrence or development of these behaviors can contribute to suboptimal weight loss.[49] The most consistent evidence to date has shown that postoperative binge eating/BED/LOC, P&N, and significant psychopathology are negative predictors of weight loss outcomes,[48,53,55] with different weight loss trajectories observed within 2 years postoperatively.[48] Specifically, approximately 65% of patients with weight regain report problematic eating behaviors,[48] and higher levels of impulsiveness are believed to play a role.[49] Thus, ongoing intervention and monitoring are needed in the postoperative period.[55] As discussed in a review by Sheets and colleagues,[55] however, positive predictors of weight loss outcomes were found among a sample of more than 2000 LABS participants (from baseline to 3-years postsurgery) who stopped eating when they felt full, stopped eating continuously throughout the day, and engaged in self-weighing; they had 14% greater weight loss than those who made no positive changes.

Eating Disorders After Bariatric Surgery

Although less common, it is increasingly recognized that a small subset of patients are diagnosed with eating disorders post–bariatric surgery.[15,57] Research indicates that traditional eating disorders, such as AN and BN, can occur after bariatric surgery and in some cases patients present for treatment with low BMIs and significant medical comorbidities, although other patients may not have a critically low BMI but nonetheless have lost excessive weight, have medical evidence of starvation, and meet current criteria for AN, which do not stipulate the necessity of a low body weight if other criteria are met.[15,57] There are no prevalence or incidence data yet available on such outcomes.

TREATMENT OF THESE EATING PROBLEMS
Presurgery

A critical component of the presurgical psychological evaluation is to identify patients with significant untreated psychopathology, including BED. An appropriate intervention should be considered (ie, referral for psychotherapy and/or psychotropic medication), but generally such interventions should be deferred until after surgery.[41] For example, nonbariatric patients meeting *DSM-5* criteria for BED typically are referred for cognitive behavior therapy (CBT), the first-line, evidence-based treatment of BED,[64] which focuses on normalization of eating patterns, reduction of binge eating,[21] and improvement in mood symptoms rather than addressing weight loss, which rarely results from such an intervention.[21] Some bariatric programs have developed brief, group CBT protocols to treat binge eating prior to surgery and found that patients with BED who completed the group improved on binge-eating scores such that they no longer met criteria for BED before surgery.[65] Antidepressants or stimulant medications also can be used in lieu of or as an adjunct to psychotherapy. BED should not be regarded, however, as a contraindication to bariatric surgery, because some patients experience a remission of BED with surgery and progress normally. Also, most bariatric surgery candidates are significantly impaired psychologically, socially, and medically, and delaying surgery for an extended time is rarely warranted.

Postsurgery

It has been well documented that problematic eating behaviors pose the greatest threat to meaningful and sustained weight loss, and that a new onset or recurrence of such behaviors (ie, LOC eating) can occur within 12 months or earlier after surgery,[50] which can result in less weight loss at long-term follow-up. This suggests the need to monitor problematic eating and intervene earlier,[48,53] which aligns with researchers who suggest the best time to target behaviors like LOC eating and clinically significant depressive symptoms is as soon as possible once they manifest postsurgery, when patient investment in treatment[38] is high and patients are motivated to succeed.[66]

Treatment of postoperative eating disorders is, again, usually CBT. Inpatient or treatment may be necessary, however, for those who develop AN or BN. Medications are typically are used for depression and adjunctive for BN and BED. The focus of CBT remains on normalizing eating patterns but topics may include issues pertaining to adjustments in foods eaten, vitamins taken, relationships, and body image, which may not have been thoroughly considered presurgery.[67]

Postsurgery treatments have used both individual and group-based CBT[66,67] and others have incorporated motivational enhancement strategies,[68] which can result in a reduction in LOC or binge-eating symptoms, increased self-efficacy, and enhanced weight loss.

ACKNOWLEDGMENTS

C.S. Brode was supported by the National Institute of General Medical Sciences, U54GM104942. The content is solely the responsibility of the authors and does not necessarily represent the official views of the NIH. J.E. Mitchell was supported by Grants U01 DK066471, UO1 DK07249, RO1 DK084979, RO1 AA022336, R01 DK80020, and R01 DK112585 from the National Institutes of Health.

REFERENCES

1. Hales CM, Fryar CD, Carroll MD, et al. Trends in obesity and severe obesity prevalence in US youth and adults by sex and age, 2007-2008 to 2015-2016. JAMA 2018;319(16):1723–5.
2. Carlsson LM, Peltonen M, Ahlin S, et al. Bariatric surgery and prevention of type 2 diabetes in Swedish obese subjects. N Engl J Med 2012;367(8):695–704.
3. Ohishi M. Hypertension with diabetes mellitus: physiology and pathology. Hypertens Res 2018;41(6):389.
4. Saklayen MG. The global epidemic of the metabolic syndrome. Curr Hypertens Rep 2018;20(2):12.
5. Winocour P. Diabetes and chronic kidney disease: an increasingly common multimorbid disease in need of a paradigm shift in care. Diabet Med 2018;35(3):300–5.
6. Courcoulas AP, King WC, Belle SH, et al. Seven-year weight trajectories and health outcomes in the Longitudinal Assessment of Bariatric Surgery (LABS) study. JAMA Surg 2018;153(5):427–34.
7. Sjöström L, Gummesson A, Sjöström CD, et al. Effects of bariatric surgery on cancer incidence in obese patients in Sweden (Swedish Obese Subjects Study): a prospective, controlled intervention trial. Lancet Oncol 2009;10(7):653–62.
8. Sjöström L, Peltonen M, Jacobson P, et al. Bariatric surgery and long-term cardiovascular events. JAMA 2012;307(1):56–65.
9. Fouladi F, Mitchell JE, Wonderlich JA, et al. The contributing role of bile acids to metabolic improvements after obesity and metabolic surgery. Obes Surg 2016;26(10):2492–502.
10. Allison KC, Wadden TA, Sarwer DB, et al. Night eating syndrome and binge eating disorder among persons seeking bariatric surgery: prevalence and related features. Obesity (Silver Spring) 2006;14(S3):77S–82S.
11. Cryan JF, Dinan TG. Mind-altering microorganisms: the impact of the gut microbiota on brain and behaviour. Nat Rev Neurosci 2012;13(10):701–12.
12. Makaronidis JM, Batterham RL. Potential mechanisms mediating sustained weight loss following Roux-en-Y gastric bypass and sleeve gastrectomy. Endocrinol Metab Clin North Am 2016;45(3):539–52.
13. Noel OF, Still CD, Argyropoulos G, et al. Bile acids, FXR, and metabolic effects of bariatric surgery. J Obes 2016;2016:4390254.
14. Sweeney TE, Morton JM. The human gut microbiome: a review of the effect of obesity and surgically induced weight loss. JAMA Surg 2013;148(6):563–9.
15. Marino JM, Ertelt TW, Lancaster K, et al. The emergence of eating pathology after bariatric surgery: a rare outcome with important clinical implications. Int J Eat Disord 2012;45(2):179–84.
16. Hudson JI, Hiripi E, Pope HG, et al. The prevalence and correlates of eating disorders in the National Comorbidity Survey Replication. Biol Psychiatry 2007;61(3):348–58.
17. Kessler RC, Chiu WT, Demler O, et al. Prevalence, severity, and comorbidity of 12-month DSM-IV disorders in the National Comorbidity Survey Replication. Arch Gen Psychiatry 2005;62(6):617–27.
18. Kalarchian MA, Marcus MD, Levine MD, et al. Psychiatric disorders among bariatric surgery candidates: relationship to obesity and functional health status. Am J Psychiatry 2007;164(2):328–34.

19. Fabricatore AN, Wadden TA, Sarwer DB, et al. Health-related quality of life and symptoms of depression in extremely obese persons seeking bariatric surgery. Obes Surg 2005;15(3):304–9.
20. Association AP. Diagnostic and statistical manual of mental disorders (DSM-5®). American Psychiatric Pub; 2013.
21. de Zwaan M. Binge eating disorder and obesity. Int J Obes 2001;25(S1):S51.
22. Friedman KE, Ashmore JA, Applegate KL. Recent experiences of weight-based stigmatization in a weight loss surgery population: psychological and behavioral correlates. Obesity (Silver Spring) 2008;16(S2):S69–74.
23. Hunte HE, Williams DR. The association between perceived discrimination and obesity in a population-based multiracial and multiethnic adult sample. Am J Public Health 2009;99(7):1285–92.
24. Macht M. How emotions affect eating: a five-way model. Appetite 2008;50(1): 1–11.
25. Colles SL, Dixon JB, O'brien PE. Loss of control is central to psychological disturbance associated with binge eating disorder. Obesity (Silver Spring) 2008;16(3): 608–14.
26. Jones-Corneille LR, Wadden TA, Sarwer DB, et al. Axis I psychopathology in bariatric surgery candidates with and without binge eating disorder: results of structured clinical interviews. Obes Surg 2012;22(3):389–97.
27. Mitchell JE, King WC, Courcoulas A, et al. Eating behavior and eating disorders in adults before bariatric surgery. Int J Eat Disord 2015;48(2):215–22.
28. Mitchell JE, Selzer F, Kalarchian MA, et al. Psychopathology before surgery in the longitudinal assessment of bariatric surgery-3 (LABS-3) psychosocial study. Surg Obes Relat Dis 2012;8(5):533–41.
29. Ambwani S, Boeka AG, Brown JD, et al. Socially desirable responding by bariatric surgery candidates during psychological assessment. Surg Obes Relat Dis 2013;9(2):300–5.
30. Engel SG, Mitchell JE, De Zwaan M, et al. Eating disorders and eating problems pre-and postbariatric surgery. Psychosocial assessment and treatment of bariatric surgery patients. Routledge; 2012. p. 99–110.
31. de Zwaan M, Mitchell JE. Eating disorders and eating behavior pre-and post-bariatric surgery. The ASMBS textbook of bariatric surgery. Springer; 2014. p. 25–32.
32. Cooper Z, Fairburn C. The eating disorder examination: a semi-structured interview for the assessment of the specific psychopathology of eating disorders. Int J Eat Disord 1987;6(1):1–8.
33. First M, Williams J, Karg R, et al. Structured clinical interview for DSM-5 disorders, clinician version (SCID-5-CV). Arlington (VA): American Psychiatric Association; 2015.
34. Fairburn CG, Beglin SJ. Assessment of eating disorders: interview or self-report questionnaire? Int J Eat Disord 1994;16(4):363–70.
35. Stunkard AJ, Messick S. Eating inventory. Psychological Corporation; 1988.
36. Colles SL, Dixon JB, O'brien PE. Grazing and loss of control related to eating: two high-risk factors following bariatric surgery. Obesity (Silver Spring) 2008;16(3): 615–22.
37. de Zwaan M, Hilbert A, Swan-Kremeier L, et al. Comprehensive interview assessment of eating behavior 18–35 months after gastric bypass surgery for morbid obesity. Surg Obes Relat Dis 2010;6(1):79–85.
38. Müller A, Mitchell JE, Sondag C, et al. Psychiatric aspects of bariatric surgery. Curr Psychiatry Rep 2013;15(10):397.

39. Conceição EM, Crosby R, Mitchell JE, et al. Picking or nibbling: frequency and associated clinical features in bulimia nervosa, anorexia nervosa, and binge eating disorder. Int J Eat Disord 2013;46(8):815–8.
40. Saunders R. "Grazing": a high-risk behavior. Obes Surg 2004;14(1):98–102.
41. Sogg S. Assessment of bariatric surgery candidates: e Clinical Interview. Psychosocial assessment and treatment of bariatric surgery patients. Routledge; 2012. p. 27–48.
42. Allison KC, Lundgren JD, O'Reardon JP, et al. The night eating questionnaire (NEQ): psychometric properties of a measure of severity of the night eating syndrome. Eat Behav 2008;9(1):62–72.
43. O'reardon JP, Ringel BL, Dinges DF, et al. Circadian eating and sleeping patterns in the night eating syndrome. Obes Res 2004;12(11):1789–96.
44. de Zwaan M, Marschollek M, Allison KC. The night eating syndrome (NES) in bariatric surgery patients. Eur Eat Disord Rev 2015;23(6):426–34.
45. Hachem A, Brennan L. Quality of life outcomes of bariatric surgery: a systematic review. Obes Surg 2016;26(2):395–409.
46. Karlsson J, Sjöström L, Sullivan M. Swedish obese subjects (SOS)–an intervention study of obesity. Two-year follow-up of health-related quality of life (HRQL) and eating behavior after gastric surgery for severe obesity. Int J Obes 1998; 22(2):113.
47. Kolotkin RL, Crosby RD, Gress RE, et al. Two-year changes in health-related quality of life in gastric bypass patients compared with severely obese controls. Surg Obes Relat Dis 2009;5(2):250–6.
48. Conceição EM, Mitchell JE, Pinto-Bastos A, et al. Stability of problematic eating behaviors and weight loss trajectories after bariatric surgery: a longitudinal observational study. Surg Obes Relat Dis 2017;13(6):1063–70.
49. Conceição E, Mitchell JE, Vaz AR, et al. The presence of maladaptive eating behaviors after bariatric surgery in a cross sectional study: importance of picking or nibbling on weight regain. Eat Behav 2014;15(4):558–62.
50. White MA, Kalarchian MA, Masheb RM, et al. Loss of control over eating predicts outcomes in bariatric surgery: a prospective 24-month follow-up study. J Clin Psychiatry 2010;71(2):175.
51. Kalarchian MA, King WC, Devlin MJ, et al. Psychiatric disorders and weight change in a prospective study of bariatric surgery patients: a 3-year follow-up. Psychosom Med 2016;78(3):373.
52. Kofman MD, Lent MR, Swencionis C. Maladaptive eating patterns, quality of life, and weight outcomes following gastric bypass: results of an Internet survey. Obesity (Silver Spring) 2010;18(10):1938–43.
53. Meany G, Conceição E, Mitchell JE. Binge eating, binge eating disorder and loss of control eating: effects on weight outcomes after bariatric surgery. Eur Eat Disord Rev 2014;22(2):87–91.
54. Sarwer DB, Wadden TA, Moore RH, et al. Preoperative eating behavior, postoperative dietary adherence, and weight loss after gastric bypass surgery. Surg Obes Relat Dis 2008;4(5):640–6.
55. Sheets CS, Peat CM, Berg KC, et al. Post-operative psychosocial predictors of outcome in bariatric surgery. Obes Surg 2015;25(2):330–45.
56. Toussi R, Fujioka K, Coleman KJ. Pre-and postsurgery behavioral compliance, patient health, and postbariatric surgical weight loss. Obesity (Silver Spring) 2009;17(5):996–1002.
57. Conceição E, Orcutt M, Mitchell J, et al. Eating disorders after bariatric surgery: a case series. Int J Eat Disord 2013;46(3):274–9.

58. Jumbe S, Hamlet C, Meyrick J. Psychological aspects of bariatric surgery as a treatment for obesity. Curr Obes Rep 2017;6(1):71–8.
59. Pinto TF, de Bruin PFC, de Bruin VMS, et al. Effects of bariatric surgery on night eating and depressive symptoms: a prospective study. Surg Obes Relat Dis 2017;13(6):1057–62.
60. Sarwer DB, Steffen KJ. Quality of life, body image and sexual functioning in bariatric surgery patients. Eur Eat Disord Rev 2015;23(6):504–8.
61. Herpertz S, Müller A, Burgmer R, et al. Health-related quality of life and psychological functioning 9 years after restrictive surgical treatment for obesity. Surg Obes Relat Dis 2015;11(6):1361–70.
62. Faulconbridge LF, Wadden TA, Thomas JG, et al. Changes in depression and quality of life in obese individuals with binge eating disorder: bariatric surgery versus lifestyle modification. Surg Obes Relat Dis 2013;9(5):790–6.
63. de Zwaan M, Lancaster KL, Mitchell JE, et al. Health-related quality of life in morbidly obese patients: effect of gastric bypass surgery. Obes Surg 2002;12(6):773–80.
64. Fairburn CG, Wilson GT, Schleimer K. Binge eating: nature, assessment, and treatment. New York: Guilford Press; 1993.
65. Ashton K, Drerup M, Windover A, et al. Brief, four-session group CBT reduces binge eating behaviors among bariatric surgery candidates. Surg Obes Relat Dis 2009;5(2):257–62.
66. LaHaise K, Mitchell J. Next Step, a bariatric psychological aftercare program. Psychosocial assessment and treatment of bariatric surgery patients. New York: Taylor & Francis; 2012. p. 231–40.
67. Saunders R. Post-surgery group therapy for gastric bypass patients. Obes Surg 2004;14(8):1128–31.
68. Stewart KE, Olbrisch ME, Bean MK. Back on track: confronting post-surgical weight gain. Bariatr Nurs Surg Patient Care 2010;5(2):179–85.

Involuntary Treatment and Quality of Life

Terry Carney, PhD(Mon), LLB (Hons), Dip Crim(Melb)[a],*, Joel Yager, MD[b],
Sarah Maguire, MA, DCP, PhD[c], Stephen William Touyz, BSc (Cape Town), PhD (Cape Town)[d]

KEYWORDS

- Anorexia nervosa • Involuntary treatment • Quality of life • Human rights

KEY POINTS

- Involuntary treatment is indicated for only a small proportion of persons experiencing life-threatening, unresponsive anorexia nervosa.
- Involuntary treatment may be contraindicated or futile for some persons with severe and enduring anorexia nervosa.
- Anorexia nervosa can have a profound effect across many domains of life.
- Patients with severe and enduring anorexia nervosa have impairments in quality of life equal to those with depression or schizophrenia.

INTRODUCTION

Involuntary treatment of anorexia nervosa (AN) poses many clinical, medicolegal, human rights, and ethical issues, as well as personal and familial challenges for the individual requiring care. From the perspective of care providers, the clinical challenge is in determining the circumstances warranting an intervention that is not requested by their client, may jeopardize the therapeutic relationship, and can potentially cause great distress for the client and carers, for a condition arguably carrying the highest psychiatric mortality rates. This is further complicated by the need to weigh evidence of the efficacy of competing treatments. The medicolegal challenge is navigating the complex conditions for invoking compulsory treatment authority and choosing between any alternative routes provided. The human rights challenge is that the Convention on the Rights of Persons with Disabilities is interpreted by its monitoring committee as ruling out retention or use of laws that override or displace a person's

[a] School of Law, The University of Sydney, New Law School Building, Eastern Avenue, New South Wales 2006, Australia; [b] Department of Psychiatry, University of Colorado School of Medicine, 13001 East 17th Place (Fitzsimons Building), MC A011-04, Aurora, CO 80045, USA; [c] InsideOut Institute, Charles Perkins Centre, University of Sydney, D17, New South Wales 2006, Australia; [d] School of Psychology and Inside Out Institute, University of Sydney, Brain Mind Centre, Room 321, 94 Mallett Street, Camperdown, New South Wales 2050, Australia
* Corresponding author.
E-mail address: Terry.carney@sydney.edu.au

Psychiatr Clin N Am 42 (2019) 299–307
https://doi.org/10.1016/j.psc.2019.01.011
0193-953X/19/© 2019 Elsevier Inc. All rights reserved.

Abbreviations	
AN	anorexia nervosa
BMI	body mass index

legal capacity to decide on treatment; the ethical challenges include balancing and applying standard bioethical principles and addressing issues of treatment futility and respect for individual autonomy. All of these challenges raise important issues of quality of life, and are heightened for the subset of persons with severe and enduring AN, a taxonomic term distilled from clinical descriptions of people with AN who have had a long and severe course of illness.[1]

THE CLINICAL CHALLENGE

Although there is considerable support for resorting to civil committal powers to coerce selected AN patients into treatment,[2] there is an ongoing debate about the specific characteristics of the group for whom this measure is justified and about when a patient should be permitted to decline a treatment, where refusal is likely to result in their death.[3–5]

Evidence-Based Treatment Decisions

The paucity of evidence that exists to help guide clinical decisions is based on poor quality studies. The literature is limited to several case series that compare relatively small numbers of patients hospitalized involuntarily, with voluntary patients seen in the same facilities over similar periods of time, and some interview-based research studying individuals who have had experience with and have subsequent opinions about coercive treatment. Optimistically, these studies generally show that short-term weight restoration outcomes for patients subject to compulsory hospitalizations are comparable with those hospitalized on a voluntary basis. For the most part, these limited case series are buttressed by anecdotes underscoring the fact that some of the patients were "saved" and "turned around" by being placed on involuntary treatment. However, where follow-up data are available, they also show that longer term outcomes for those hospitalized involuntarily is considerably worse than for voluntary hospitalized patients, which is not surprising given that involuntarily hospitalized patients are often sicker, have greater comorbidities, and are almost always less motivated to seek care after discharge from compulsory hospital treatment. Although some anecdotal cases also describe patients who die despite being placed into involuntary treatment, few of these cases appear in print, again not surprising, given that few clinicians are motivated and willing to publish what they and others might perceive to be treatment failures. Although numerous discussions of various legal, moral, ethical, and clinical issues are available, only a few data-based studies provide possible guidance.

Ramsay and colleagues[6] reported on 81 patients admitted to the Eating Disorders Unit at the Maudsley Hospital under Britain's Mental Health Act for compulsory treatment (16% of all admissions to the unit). Before their index admission, 7 had been previously involuntarily admitted once, 4 detained twice, 3 detained 3 times, and 1 detained 4 times. These involuntarily admitted patients were matched and compared with 81 patients admitted voluntarily during the same time periods. Admission data on patients admitted on involuntary versus voluntary status included numerous measures on which the 2 groups did not differ significantly; for example, respectively, average ages were 26.2 versus 25.4 years, mean length of illness 8.2 versus 7.6 years; mean admission body mass index (BMI) 14.2 versus 14.3; history of binge eating 40.7%

versus 44.4%; history of purging 50.6% versus 44.4%; and presence of comorbidity, 44.4% versus 30.9%. Statistically significant differences were seen, respectively, for childhood physical or sexual abuse (24.1% vs 10.1%); histories of self-harm (59.3% vs 33.3%); and number of previous admissions (mean 3.3 vs 1.8). Notably, the length of admission was significantly longer for the involuntary patient group (mean 113 days vs 88 days), but the discharge BMIs were very similar (mean 18.7 vs 18.5), showing that with some effort comparable short-term outcomes could be achieved, at least with respect to weight restoration. At an average follow-up of 5.7 years, data were obtained from the National Health Service Registry on patients in this group who had died and their causes of death. At follow-up, 12.7% of the involuntary group had died (10 of 79 for whom data were available), compared with only 2.6% of the voluntary group—discouraging, but not surprising. One death in the involuntary group was attributed to "misadventure"; the others were attributed to a variety of cardiac and pulmonary causes and to AN. A 2015 publication[7] updated follow-up data on mortality in this cohort, by which point a total of 27 of the 162 patients had died (26 of 155 females; average age at death, 37.7 years), 5 by suicide with 18 of the deaths directly attributed to AN and its complications. Subsequent to the initial follow-up, an additional 7 patients in the compulsory group and 8 patients in the noncompulsory group died. Overall standardized mortality ratios for compulsory and noncompulsory patients, respectively, were 7.65 and 4.59. Overall, the risk of premature death was considerably greater in the initial 10 years of follow-up compared with later on. The authors concluded that compulsory treatment itself seemingly has little effect on the longer term mortality rate, including suicide.

In a similar study of 397 patients admitted to the University of Iowa eating disorders unit over a period of 7 years, 66 (16.6%) of whom were admitted through involuntary legal commitment (60 females and 6 males), Watson and colleagues[8] also found relatively few clinical differences between voluntary and involuntary admissions. The involuntarily admitted patients averaged 24 years of age, 28 (42%) were diagnosed with AN, 18 (27%) with bulimia nervosa, and the remaining 20 (31%) with an eating disorder not otherwise specified. On average, these patients were not as ill as those described in the Ramsay and colleagues study. The mean length of illness among the involuntary patients was 96.8 weeks (standard deviation, 75.8 weeks), the average BMI on admission was 17.4, and the average BMI at discharge was 20.5. The overwhelming majority had 5 or fewer previous hospitalizations, but a minority (9 of 386) had 10 or more prior hospitalizations. Among the involuntary patients, 47% had comorbid diagnoses of depression and 29% of substance abuse. As in the Ramsay and colleagues study, involuntary patients required longer hospitalizations than voluntary patients (56.7 days vs 40.6 days), and by discharge averaged greater weight gain than voluntary patients (18.8 pounds compared with 13.9 pounds). The short-term outcomes with regard to weights were comparable: focusing only on the involuntarily hospitalized patients with AN, by discharge their average mean weight compared with matched population control weights was 90.5% versus 91.2% for voluntarily admitted patients. Anecdotally, the authors note that by the time of discharge many of the involuntarily admitted patients acknowledged recognizing and endorsing the need for treatment. No long-term follow-up data were included in this study.

More recently, Westmoreland and Mehler[9] compared the course and outcome of 109 patients admitted under involuntary certification to the Eating Recovery Center in Denver, Colorado, from 2012 to 2016. Of these, 31% successfully completed treatment and 42% returned for a further episode of care. Of note, 24% of the certifications were terminated because involuntary treatment was not found to be helpful. Conclusions supported by these data are that patients with AN who are the most medically ill often require involuntary treatment. In addition, although many patients who were certified successfully completed treatment, involuntary treatment was not felt to be helpful approximately 25% of the time. In these instances, treating psychiatrists asked that the certifications be discontinued because in their estimation patients had "reached maximum benefit under certification" (opining that patients would derive no additional benefits from further treatment, and that further treatment would likely do more harm than good). In their experience, civil commitment may not be helpful when patients repeatedly "abscond," are unwilling to graduate from forced tube feeding to voluntary tube feeding and then to eating meals, have failed multiple previous treatment programs, are of older age, and meet criteria for a harm reduction model, palliative care, or hospice care.[9] This group anticipates that additional study may permit refinement of criteria to define which patients are most suitable—or unsuitable—for involuntary commitment and treatment.[10]

Although not specifically studying people with the illness admitted on involuntary legal status, the results reported by Guarda and colleagues[11] might also inform discussions concerning the coercive persuasion of hospitalized people with the illness with eating disorders. In their study of 139 patients admitted "voluntarily" to Johns Hopkins University's eating disorders programs, many felt that they were coerced into treatment. The patients' average age was 25.2 years, 55% had AN (34% the restricting subtype of AN and 21% AN with bulimia nervosa), 30% bulimia nervosa, and the remainder an eating disorder not otherwise specified. More perceived coercion was reported among the 35 patients under age 18 than among the 104 adults. Thirty of the adults did not endorse needing admission, but by 2 weeks into hospitalizations 17 changed their minds and agreed that they needed hospitalization. No differences were seen between the restricting subtype of AN and AN with bulimia nervosa, although the small sample size may have obscured differences that might be seen in larger samples. Unfortunately, the absence of data in this report on the duration of illness, previous treatment, comorbidities, and other pertinent factors limits what we might infer from this study with respect to AN, a view consistent with other studies.[12]

To summarize, these studies suggest that, with extra time and effort, the short-term weight restoration of patients hospitalized involuntarily for AN might be comparable with that seen in voluntarily admitted patients, that a reasonable number of people might actually come around to acknowledge their need for treatment, and that some might even be thankful (or at least tell their caregivers that they were thankful) for the fact that they were treated, even against their will. However, the literature contains a paucity of detailed descriptions differentiating those involuntarily treated people who benefited in both the short term and the long term from those who rapidly relapsed and even succumbed. The many gaps in knowledge suggest that large, multisite studies on treatment-refusing people with AN (inclusive of those who feel coerced) will be required if we are ever to be able to make clinical decisions based on concrete evidence rather than, at best, informed anecdote and whim.

THE MEDICOLEGAL AND HUMAN RIGHTS CHALLENGE
A Varied Mosaic of Legal Avenues for Involuntary Treatment

The age of the person requiring care is a factor in medicolegal considerations. Involuntary treatment of an adolescent with AN is governed by the same laws as cover other important decisions. Parental consent is required at common law, subject in many of the 53 Commonwealth countries to a 'mature minor' exception, empowering a decision to be made by someone of an age and maturity of mind to be able to understand and weigh the consequences of the particular question (the Gillick principle[13]). In North America, parental consent is more strongly entrenched in common law, but some states in the United States have legislated age-specific exceptions for older adolescents, whereas in countries such as Australia, provision is made for adult guardianship laws to apply before adulthood (usually at 16).[14]

Jurisdictions vary in their legal requirements for coercive treatment. In a number of jurisdictions, the authorizations for involuntary committal to care and the authority to provide involuntary treatment while committed are dealt with separately. Although involuntary committal is commonly available for both adults and young people under mental health laws globally, only some jurisdictions authorize treatment of involuntary patients without their consent.[15] In jurisdictions (such as much of North America) requiring separate authorization to actively treat involuntary in-patients, treatment without consent hinges on the patient exhibiting a lack of capacity to give informed consent at common law. In jurisdictions such as England and Wales, which have enacted legislation defining capacity (and authorizing the treatment of persons lacking capacity), involuntary treatment for AN is seen as an issue of legal capacity.[16] In North America, civil commitment is generally available under mental health civil commitment legislation,[17] whereas in Australian jurisdictions such as New South Wales and Victoria, there is a choice between mental health and adult guardianship legislation[18] and, within mental health, between involuntary residential and involuntary community treatment orders. Provisions enabling citizens to make or enforce so-called advance directives authorizing the form of any future treatment (including involuntary treatment) exist in many jurisdictions,[17,19] although they are apparently infrequently executed by people with AN.

Variable Take-Up of Legal Options

Having an available legal avenue for involuntary treatment is one issue, but its utilization is quite another. Thus, civil commitment seems to be rarely used (or perhaps even contemplated) in the United States.[17,20] In Australia, where the largest jurisdictions have almost identical mental health and adult guardianship laws, Victoria relies entirely on mental health commitment laws, eschewing the use of adult guardianship found across the border in New South Wales, because to do so is seen to be contrary to the more 'empowering' philosophy of adult guardianship (which also involves interposing a guardian between the patient and the clinician).[21] Important differences exist in the form of mental health laws. Some laws empower clinicians to treat involuntarily a patient to later review, whereas others require an initial order of a legal body.[14] Much of North America relies on courts as gatekeepers, whereas Australia and Britain use multidisciplinary tribunals for the authorization and review of coercive powers. A third approach (such as in Victoria, Australia) lies in giving weight to less interventionist options, such as third-party 'support' and advance directives. In short, there is both considerable variance in the international pattern of laws regarding mental health generally[22] or AN in particular,[14] as well as some uncertainty about the boundaries of what is permissible with regard to involuntary AN management in particular countries.[23]

A Plethora of Extralegal Issues and Values in Play in Mobilizing Involuntary Treatment

For clinicians and the law alike, a major challenge in using these avenues lies in aligning clinical evidence with the underlying philosophy of the legislation (beneficent treatment in the case of mental health; last resort facilitation of impaired autonomy in the case of guardianship) and conveying clinical understandings in ways attuned to the language of and operating practice of the tribunals or courts administering the law. Rules and practices around invoking an involuntary patient status or use of coerced treatment vary a great deal from country to country, between states or regions of federations, and even between individual decision makers or panels within the same court or tribunal. These extralegal value-dependent factors cover differences in judicial philosophy (ranging from libertarian to, at best, compassionate paternalism), differences in individual temperament in emotional reactions to pleas by the person or their family, or differences in personal experience or exposure to family or friends with AN members or other psychiatric disorders. In the United States, asking a judge to place a patient on involuntary status for treatment in no way assures that the judge will side with family, friends, or professionals who are pressing the case. For example, in invoking involuntary hospitalization for a person with AN, some judges have used the mental health standard that involuntary hospitalization can be imposed if the person is "gravely disabled," defined as unable to provide herself with "food, clothing or shelter," focusing on her inability to provide herself with "food." Other judges disagree vehemently with such an interpretation. Mental health adjudication by tribunals, for its part, has been shown to also be replete with such extralegal determinants of outcomes.[15,24,25] Common law jurisdictions retaining a 'best interests' test—a criterion so open ended that it has been described as an "empty vessel" into which the perceptions or prejudices of the decision maker may be poured—also encounter disquiet about a lack of certainty, as in England and Wales, where its capacity legislation empowers judges of their Court of Protection to make often controversial decisions about whether or not to order the involuntary feeding of people with AN.[26]

CONTEMPORARY HUMAN RIGHTS, QUALITY OF LIFE, AND OTHER CHALLENGES

The monitoring committee for the Convention on the Rights of Persons with Disabilities, a convention subscribed to by most countries (the United States being a notable exception), interprets it as being incompatible with retention of involuntary treatment, adult guardianship, or other forms of substitute decision making or wardship authorities that detract from respect for legal capacity.[27] Instead, the focus is on provision of "support" to enable the person to continue making their own decisions.

Supported decision making poses considerable challenges of finding and prioritizing monetary and human resources to assist those lacking family or others willing to assume responsibility for facilitating informed decision making,[28,29] and major dilemmas where clinicians lose confidence in the judgment of family members.[14] Others have instead explored recasting legal capacity tests to be more attuned to the Convention on the Rights of Persons with Disabilities by incorporating considerations of beneficence,[30] but this still leaves a Convention on the Rights of Persons with Disabilities noncompliant finding of incapacity as one outcome, along with retaining a crude binary between intervention and no intervention. Perhaps more promising, if still fraught owing to its slipperiness, is the prospect of greater use of the many intermediate points on the gradation between autonomy and substituted/imposed decisions, from mere conversational suasion, through various forms of "leverage," and possible culmination in moral blackmail, which can be perceived as being as coercive as a formal order. Clinicians are already quite familiar with the usefulness (and risks) of such tools and are skilled in their use,[19,31] which can extend to strategic lodgment and later withdrawal of applications for legal orders such as guardianship to nudge treatment compliance.[32,33] However, much work remains before any new direction for law or clinical practice can be predicted with any confidence.

SUMMARY

The multifaceted complexity of issues centering on the involuntary treatment of those with chronic and enduring AN are daunting. There is now a general consensus that patients with AN and especially those with the more severe and enduring subtype are more likely to have high levels of disability, to be underemployed or unemployed, to be receiving welfare, and to be a significant burden to family, carers, and health fund providers.[34] It is no longer an overstatement to assert that such patients show a similar degree of impairment on measures of quality of life as those with depression or schizophrenia.[35] It is now possible to mount a cogent argument as to why a rehabilitation model of care, not too dissimilar to the ones advocated for those with schizophrenia, needs to be considered for those with a more persistent eating disorder, including highly specialized acute care when the need arises.[36] In such cases, harm minimization and improved quality of life should be prioritized and involuntary treatment should only be used judiciously.

REFERENCES

1. Broomfield C, Stedal K, Touyz S, et al. Labeling and defining severe and enduring anorexia nervosa: a systematic review and critical analysis. Int J Eat Disord 2017; 50(6):611–23.
2. Bowers WA. Civil commitment in the treatment of eating disorders and substance abuse: empirical status and ethical considerations. In: Brewerton TD, Dennis AB, editors. Eating disorders, addictions and substance use disorders. Dordrecht (Netherlands): Springer; 2014. p. 649–64.
3. Giordano S. Anorexia and refusal of life-saving treatment: the moral place of competence, suffering, and the family. Philos Psychiatry Psychol 2010;17(2): 143–54.
4. Gans M, Gunn WB. End-stage anorexia: criteria for competence to refuse treatment. In: Sisti DA, Caplan AL, Rimon-Greenspan H, editors. Applied ethics in mental health care: an interdisciplinary reader. Cambridge (MA): MIT Press; 2013. p. 91–114.
5. Lopez A, Yager J, Feinstein RE. Medical futility and psychiatry: palliative care and hospice care as a last resort in the treatment of refractory anorexia nervosa. Int J Eat Disord 2010;43(4):372–7.
6. Ramsay R, Ward A, Treasure J, et al. Compulsory treatment in anorexia nervosa. Short-term benefits and long-term mortality. Br J Psychiatry 1999;175:147–53.
7. Ward A, Ramsay R, Russell G, et al. Follow-up mortality study of compulsorily treated patients with anorexia nervosa. Int J Eat Disord 2015;48(7):860–5.
8. Watson T, Bowers W, Andersen A. Involuntary treatment of eating disorders. Am J Psychiatry 2000;157:1806–10.
9. Westmoreland P, Mehler P. Caring for patients with severe and enduring eating disorders (SEED): certification, harm reduction, palliative care, and the question of futility. J Psychiatr Pract 2016;22(4):313–20.
10. Westmoreland P, Johnson C, Stafford M, et al. Involuntary treatment of patients with life-threatening anorexia nervosa. J Am Acad Psychiatry Law 2017;45(4): 419–25.
11. Guarda AS, Pinto A, Coughlin J, et al. Perceived coercion and change in perceived need for admission in patients hospitalized for eating disorders. Am J Psychiatry 2007;164(1):108–14.
12. Griffiths R, Beumont P, Russell J, et al. The use of guardianship legislation for anorexia nervosa: a report of 15 cases. Aust N Z J Psychiatry 1997;31:525–31.

13. Cave E. Goodbye Gillick? Identifying and resolving problems with the concept of child competence. Leg Stud 2014;34(1):103–22.

14. Carney T, Tait D, Touyz S, et al. Managing anorexia nervosa: clinical, legal & social perspectives on involuntary treatment. New York: Nova Science; 2006.

15. Carney T, Tait D, Perry J, et al. Australian Mental Health Tribunals: 'Space' for fairness, freedom, protection & treatment? Sydney (Australia): Themis Press; 2011.

16. Cave E, Tan J. Severe and enduring anorexia nervosa in the England and Wales Court of Protection. International Journal of Mental Health and Capacity Law 2017;23(17):4–24.

17. Bowers W. Civil commitment in the treatment of eating disorders: practical and ethical considerations. New York: Routledge; 2018.

18. Johnson A, Schyvens M, Maloney D. Mental health: coercive treatment options for anorexia under the 'Mental Health' and 'Guardianship Acts'. LSJ: Law Society of NSW Journal 2017;37:86.

19. Tan J, Richards L. Legal and ethical issues in the treatment of really sick patients with anorexia nervosa. In: Robinson PH, Nicholls D, editors. Critical care for anorexia nervosa. Cham (Switzerland): Springer; 2015. p. 113–50.

20. Testa M, West SG. Civil commitment in the United States. Psychiatry (Edgmont) 2010;7(10):30–40.

21. Carney T, Tait D, Saunders D, et al. Institutional options in management of coercion in anorexia treatment: the antipodean experiment. Int J Law Psychiatry 2003; 26(6):647–75.

22. Gray JE, McSherry BM, O'Reilly RL, et al. Australian and Canadian mental health acts compared. Aust N Z J Psychiatry 2010;44(12):1126–31.

23. Maher C, Nwachukwu I. The challenge of managing severely ill patients with anorexia nervosa in Ireland. Ir J Psychol Med 2012;29(2):69–71.

24. Perkins E. Decision-making in mental health review tribunals. London: Policy Studies Institute; 2003.

25. Peay J. Tribunals on trial: a study of decision-making under the mental health Act 1983. Oxford (England): Clarendon Press; 1989.

26. Whiteman J. Limiting Autonomy? Mental capacity to refuse treatment in the UK. Equal Rights Review 2012;9:149–53.

27. Series L, Arstein-Kerslake A, Kamundia E. Legal capacity: a global analysis of reform trends. In: Blanck P, Flynn E, editors. Routledge handbook of disability law and human rights. London: Routledge; 2017. p. 137–55.

28. Carney T. Prioritising supported decision-making: running on empty or a basis for glacial-to-steady progress? Laws 2017;6(18):1–14.

29. Byrne M, White B, McDonald F. A new tool to assess compliance of mental health laws with the Convention on the Rights of Persons with Disabilities. Int J Law Psychiatry 2018;58:122–42.

30. Boyle S. Determining capacity: how beneficence can operate in an autonomy-focussed legal regime. Elder L.J. 2018;26(1):35–63.

31. Rathner G. A plea against compulsory treatment of anorexia nervosa patients. In: Vandereycken W, Beumont P, editors. Treating eating disorders: ethical, legal and personal issues, vol. 1. London: The Athlone Press; 1998. p. 179–215.

32. Carney T, Ingvarson M, Tait D. Constructing "control" over anorexia nervosa. In: Bennett B, Carney T, Karpin I, editors. The brave new world of health. Sydney (Australia): Federation Press; 2008. p. 182–94.

33. Carney T, Tait D, Touyz S. Coercion is coercion? Reflections on clinical trends in use of compulsion in treatment of anorexia nervosa patients. Australas Psychiatry 2007;15(5):390–5.

34. Touyz S, Le Grange D, Lacey H, et al. Treating severe and enduring anorexia nervosa: a randomized controlled trial. Psychol Med 2013;43(12):2501–11.
35. Robinson P. Severe and Enduring Eating Disorder (SEED) Management of complex presentations of anorexia and bulimia nervosa. Chichester (England): Wiley; 2009.
36. Touyz S, Hay P. Severe and enduring anorexia nervosa (SE-AN): in search of a new paradigm. J Eat Disord 2015;3(1):26.

Eating Disorder Prevention

Eric Stice, PhD[a],*, Sarah Johnson, BA[a], Roxane Turgon, MA[b]

KEYWORDS

- Eating disorders • Risk factors • Prevention programs • Implementation

KEY POINTS

- Thin-ideal internalization, body dissatisfaction, overeating, dieting, fasting, and psychosocial impairment most consistently predict onset of bulimia nervosa, binge-eating disorder, and purging disorder.
- Low body mass index and low dietary restraint predict future onset of anorexia nervosa.
- Body Project and Healthy Weight are the only prevention programs that reduce eating disorder onset and eating disorder symptoms across multiple trials and independent teams.
- Other prevention programs have shown effective in single trials.
- An important future direction is to develop prevention programs that target risk factors for anorexia nervosa.

Eating disorders affect 13% of girls and women[1] and are marked by chronicity, relapse, distress, functional impairment, and increased risk for future obesity, depression, suicide, substance abuse, and mortality. Given that 80% of individuals with eating disorders do not receive treatment,[2] a public health priority is to broadly implement eating disorder prevention programs that have been found to reduce future onset of eating disorders or eating disorder symptoms. This article summarizes risk factors that have been found to predict future onset of the various types of eating disorders, describes the evidence base for prevention programs that have reduced future eating disorder onset or eating disorder symptoms, and concludes by offering suggestions for future research on eating disorder prevention.

RISK FACTORS FOR FUTURE ONSET OF EATING DISORDERS
Anorexia Nervosa

Only 2 prospective studies used risk factors assessed at baseline to predict future onset of anorexia nervosa among individuals confirmed to be free of an eating disorder at baseline. This type of prospective design definitively establishes that the risk factors

The authors have no affiliations with or involvement in any organization or entity with any financial interest in the subject matter or materials discussed in this article.

[a] Oregon Research Institute, 1776 Millrace Drive, Eugene, OR 97403, USA; [b] University Grenoble Alpes, LIP/PC2, Universite Grenoble Alpes, BP 47, Grenoble 38040 Cedex 9, France
* Corresponding author.
E-mail address: estice@ori.org

temporally preceded onset of clinically significant eating pathology. Low body mass index (BMI), low dietary restraint, assessed with the Dutch Restrained Eating Scale predicted anorexia nervosa onset, but the authors' work has shown early puberty, perceived pressure for thinness, thin-ideal internalization, body dissatisfaction, negative affect, and social support deficits did not.[3] Similarly, in a high-risk sample of young women with body dissatisfaction, low BMI, and impaired psychosocial functioning, which reflects impaired relationships with parents, friends, and peers, predicted anorexia nervosa onset, but thin-ideal internalization, positive expectances regarding thinness, denial of the costs of pursuing the thin ideal, body dissatisfaction, weight control behaviors, dieting, overeating, fasting, excessive exercise, negative affect, and mental health care did not.[4]

Three studies assessed risk factors during a developmental period that predates the typical emergence of anorexia nervosa. These studies provide evidence of temporal precedence, but did not confirm that participants were free of an eating disorder when baseline data were collected. Vaginal instrumental delivery, cephalhematoma, premature birth, low birth weight, and cobirth correlated with anorexia nervosa onset, but maternal age at childbirth, number of overall maternal births, pregnancy complications, pregnancy hypertension, diabetes, pregnancy bleeding, preterm membrane rupture, cesarean delivery, and neonatal jaundice did not.[5] In a longitudinal study that assessed children in early and late adolescence as well as in early adulthood, childhood eating conflicts, struggles around meals, and unpleasant meals correlated with anorexia nervosa onset, whereas childhood pica, digestive problems, not eating, disinterest in food, picky eating, eating too little, and eating too slowly did not.[6] Controlling for childhood eating disorder symptoms, perfectionism, and low BMI during childhood correlated with lifetime diagnoses of anorexia nervosa, but negative affect, impulsivity, and family functioning did not.[7]

Bulimia Nervosa

Seven prospective studies examined risk factors that predicted future bulimia nervosa onset. Adolescent dieters versus nondieters showed greater future bulimia nervosa onset.[8] Weight concerns, drive for thinness, body dissatisfaction, ineffectiveness, negative affectivity, dieting, alcohol use, and lower interoceptive awareness predicted bulimia nervosa onset, but perfectionism, maturity fears, interpersonal distrust, and BMI did not.[9] Dieting and psychiatric problems predicted bulimia nervosa onset, but peer dieting, daily exercise, and parental separation did not.[10] Dieting and fasting predicted bulimia nervosa onset.[11] Social pressure to be thin and body dissatisfaction predicted bulimia nervosa onset over follow-up, but thin-ideal internalization, dieting, negative affect, and depressive symptoms did not.[12] Elevated BMI, social pressure for thinness, thin-ideal internalization, dieting, negative affect, social support deficits, and early puberty predicted bulimia nervosa onset, but body dissatisfaction did not.[3] Thin-ideal internalization, positive expectances from thinness, denial of the costs of pursuing the thin ideal, body dissatisfaction, dieting, overeating, fasting, negative affect, impaired social functioning, and mental health care predicted bulimia nervosa onset in a high-risk sample of body-dissatisfied young women, but weight control behaviors, excessive exercise, and BMI did not.[4]

Two studies assessed risk factors during a developmental period that predates the typical emergence of bulimia nervosa, although neither study confirmed participants were free of an eating disorder at baseline. Eating too little during childhood correlated with bulimia nervosa onset, but childhood pica, digestive problems, eating conflicts, not eating, disinterest in food, picky eating, struggles around eating, eating too slowly, and unpleasant meals did not.[6] Controlling for childhood eating disorder symptoms, negative affect during childhood correlated with lifetime diagnoses of bulimia nervosa, but perfectionism, BMI, impulsivity, and family functioning did not.[7]

Binge-Eating Disorder

Two studies investigated baseline factors that predicted future binge-eating disorder onset. Social pressure for thinness predicted binge-eating disorder onset, but thin-ideal internalization, body dissatisfaction, dieting, and negative affect/depressive symptoms did not.[12] Thin-ideal internalization, positive expectances regarding thinness, body dissatisfaction, dieting, overeating, negative affect, impaired social functioning, and mental health care predicted binge-eating disorder onset in a high-risk sample of body-dissatisfied young women, but denial of the costs of pursuing the thin ideal, weight control behaviors, fasting, excessive exercise, and BMI did not.[4]

Purging Disorder

Two studies investigated baseline risk factors that predicted future onset of purging disorder. Thin-ideal internalization, body dissatisfaction, and dieting predicted purging disorder onset, but social pressure to be thin, negative affect, and depressive symptoms did not.[12] Thin-ideal internalization, positive expectances about thinness, denial of the costs of pursuing the thin ideal, body dissatisfaction, dieting, fasting, overeating, excessive exercise, negative affect, impaired social functioning, and mental health care predicted purging disorder onset in a high-risk sample of body-dissatisfied young women, but weight control behaviors and BMI did not.[4]

Risk Factors for Onset of Any Eating Disorder

Eight prospective studies assessed baseline risk factors that predict future onset of any eating disorder. Drive for thinness and dieting predicted onset of any eating disorder, but BMI, body dissatisfaction, perfectionism, ineffectiveness, interpersonal distrust, interoceptive awareness, psychiatric symptoms, family psychiatric disorders, family conflicts, and parental obesity did not.[13] Low self-esteem, body dissatisfaction, low family social support, and escape/avoidance coping predicted onset of any eating disorder, but BMI at baseline did not.[14] Social pressure to be thin and body dissatisfaction predicted onset of any eating disorder, but substance use, parental pressure for thinness, social support, negative life events, and school performance did not.[15] Among a high-risk sample of young women who endorsed weight-concerns, receiving negative comments about eating from siblings, coaches, and teachers; body dissatisfaction; thin-ideal internalization; parental overweight; alcohol use; and history of major depression and panic disorder predicted onset of any eating disorder, but receiving negative comments about weight, dieting, interoceptive awareness, perfectionism, emotional eating, low-self-esteem, BMI, social support deficits, social impairment, family eating disorders, parental depression and substance abuse disorders, coping strategies, anxiety disorders, depressive symptoms, emotional and sexual abuse, and negative life events did not.[16] Perceived pressure to be thin, thin-ideal internalization, body dissatisfaction, dieting, and negative affectivity predicted onset of any eating disorder, but BMI did not.[17] Self-objectification, thin-ideal internalization, body dissatisfaction, dieting, and negative affectivity predicted futures onset of any eating disorder.[2]

Four studies assessed risk factors during a developmental period that predates the typical emergence of eating disorders, although these studies did not confirm that participants were free of an eating disorder at baseline. Physical neglect and sexual abuse during childhood were correlated with onset of any eating disorder.[18] Parental separation, solitary eating, and reading teen magazines predicted onset of any eating disorder, but hours of television viewing, family stressful life events, and family history of psychiatric disorders did not.[19] Controlling for initial symptoms, low parental support negative affect, and body dissatisfaction correlated with future eating disorder diagnosis, but self-esteem, socioeconomic status, eating disorders in siblings, dysfunctional family dynamics, low peer social support, self-injury, and suicidal ideation/attempts did not.[20] Female gender, parental perception of excess body fat in the child, social withdrawal, and family stress correlated with onset of any eating disorder except anorexia nervosa, but self-esteem, body dissatisfaction, self-efficacy, intelligence, social problems, externalizing behaviors, depressive symptoms, alcohol use, paternal or maternal BMI, maternal drug use, and maternal psychiatric problems did not.[21,22] Some of these findings are based on a single study and more work needs to be pursued in this important area.

In sum, body dissatisfaction, negative affect, thin-ideal internalization, perceived pressure for thinness, dieting, and family support deficits most consistently predicted any eating disorder. Pursuit of the thin beauty ideal, body dissatisfaction, overeating, dieting, fasting, and psychosocial impairment predicted onset of bulimia nervosa, binge-eating disorder, and purging disorder. These findings suggest that prevention programs should (1) seek to reduce these risk factors and (2) target individuals with elevated levels of these risk factors in selective prevention programs. As reviewed subsequently, many of the prevention programs that have decreased eating disorder onset and symptoms focus on reducing pursuit of the thin beauty ideal, body dissatisfaction, overeating, and unhealthy weight control behaviors. A key finding from these risk factor studies, however, is that most of these risk factors have not predicted anorexia nervosa onset. Curiously, low BMI and low dietary restraint predicted future anorexia nervosa onset, suggesting that individuals who are constitutionally thin or thin because of some other factors, such as elevated satiety signaling or lower hunger signaling of gut peptides, are at risk for anorexia nervosa. These findings imply that current eating disorder prevention programs may be ineffective in preventing anorexia nervosa onset and that it might be necessary to target low-weight adolescent girls with prevention programs that promote healthy weight gain. Another unexpected finding was that only impaired psychosocial functioning predicted future onset of all types of eating disorders. Current etiologic theories of eating pathology do not implicate impaired psychosocial functioning. Risk factor findings imply, however, that a prevention program that improved psychosocial functioning among young women with impairments in this domain might effectively prevent the full spectrum of eating disorders, rather than only those involving binge-eating and compensatory behaviors. Theoretically, impaired psychosocial functioning might prompt pursuit of the thin beauty ideal as a way of achieving greater social acceptance.

EVIDENCE-BASED EATING DISORDER PREVENTION PROGRAMS

Although dozens of eating disorder prevention programs have been evaluated, most have not reduced future onset of eating disorders, the ultimate goal of prevention programs, or initial eating disorder symptoms, a reasonable objective of selective prevention programs that target high-risk individuals. This article describes eating disorder prevention programs that have produced effects for 1 or both of these key outcomes. Many of the prevention programs that were evaluated were educational in nature but were not found to prevent future eating disorder onset, which prompted a focus on reducing risk factors that had been found to increase risk for onset of eating disorders (eg, thin-ideal internalization and body dissatisfaction).

Body Project

The Body Project produced significantly greater reductions in eating disorder symptoms than the Healthy Weight eating disorder prevention program, an expressive writing comparison condition, and assessment-only controls and produced significantly greater reductions in future eating disorder onset over 3-year follow-up relative to assessment-only controls in a large efficacy trial.[23,24] In the Body Project, adolescent girls and young women discuss the negative effects of pursuing the thin beauty ideal in a variety of verbal, written, and behavioral exercises, which theoretically generate cognitive dissonance, an uncomfortable psychological state that motives people to align their attitudes with their publicly displayed behavior.[25] That is, when people discuss the negative effects of pursuing the thin ideal, it prompts a reduction in pursuit of the thin ideal because people seek to maintain consistency between their behaviors and their cognitions. The Body Project has been found to produce reductions in these outcomes for adolescent girls, young women, and older women, including both heterosexual and nonheterosexual women, as well as for homosexual and heterosexual men.[26,27] It has also been shown effective for a variety of ethnic groups.[28,29] Reduced thin-ideal internalization putatively decreases body dissatisfaction, unhealthy dietary behaviors, negative affect, and eating disorder symptoms. The Body Project also produced significantly greater reductions in eating disorder symptoms in efficacy trials conducted by others.[30–33] Participants randomized to versions of the Body Project designed to maximize versus minimize dissonance-induction showed greater eating disorder symptom reductions,[34,35] providing a critical test of the intervention theory for this prevention program. Young women who completed the Body Project also showed a greater reduction in reward region responsivity to thin models compared with educational brochure controls,[36] providing further support for the intervention theory for this program. The evidence that the Body Project reduced objectively measured neural response likewise reduces concerns that effects are the product of demand characteristics. Furthermore, the fact that the Body Project has produced effects in trials conducted by several independent teams is vital because many findings do not replicate.

Effectiveness trials have confirmed that the Body Project produces reductions in the same outcomes when delivered by high school and college counselors under ecologically valid conditions,[37,38] although in these 2 effectiveness trials the Body Project did not significantly reduce future eating disorder onset. Other effectiveness trials indicate that the Body Project produces reductions in eating disorder symptoms when delivered by undergraduate peer educators.[39–43] It is important that the Internet-based version of the Body Project did produce significant reductions in eating disorder symptoms at post-test and 6-month follow-ups,[43] because this is a rare effect for an Internet-based eating disorder prevention programs.

Healthy Weight

The Healthy Weight prevention program reduced eating disorder symptoms, relative to expressive writing and assessment-only controls; future eating disorder onset over 3-year follow-up, relative to assessment-only controls; BMI gain, relative to the Body Project, expressive-writing controls, and assessment-only controls; and obesity onset, relative to assessment-only controls in a large efficacy trial.[23,24] In this group-based intervention, young women with body image concerns make small, permanent healthy changes to dietary intake and exercise that bring caloric intake and expenditure into balance, which should reduce weight gain and risk for eating pathology. The trials that evaluated this prevention program have included adolescent girls, young women, and middle-aged women from a broad range of ethnic groups, although research has not expressly tested whether it is equally effective for participants from different age groups, different ethnic groups, and individuals with different sexual orientations. A refined version of Healthy Weight resulted in greater eating disorder symptom reductions, a 60% reduction in eating disorder onset over 2-year follow-up versus educational brochure controls, and less BMI gain through 6-month follow-up in a second efficacy trial.[44,45] An expanded 6-session version of Healthy Weight produced greater reductions in eating disorder symptoms and BMI than the cognitive reappraisal–based Minding Health obesity prevention program as well as greater reductions in body fat and eating disorder symptoms than educational video controls in another efficacy trial.[46]

A 6-hour dissonance-based version of the Healthy Weight intervention, referred to as Project Health, that added verbal and written exercises to create dissonance regarding unhealthy lifestyle behaviors that contribute to excess weight gain, produced significantly smaller increases in BMI through 2-year follow-up versus participants who completed the original Healthy Weight intervention lacking the dissonance-induction activities and obesity education video controls in an effectiveness trial involving both young women and men.[43] Project Health participants also showed significantly less overweight/obesity onset over 2-year follow-up versus Healthy Weight participants and controls—41% and 43% reductions in overweight/obesity onset versus these comparison conditions, respectively. Critically, Healthy Weight and Project Health participants also showed significantly greater reductions in eating disorder symptom than educational video controls through 2-year follow-up. Furthermore, Healthy Weight and Project Health participants showed marginally lower eating disorder onset over 2-year follow-up than educational video controls (3% and 3% vs 9%, respectively). To the authors' knowledge, Project Health and Healthy Weight are the only prevention programs to reduce both eating disorder symptoms and eating disorder onset as well as BMI gain and onset of overweight/obesity.

Student Bodies

Although the Student Bodies eating disorder prevention program did not produce a significant main effect for future eating disorder onset, it is described in this article because it reduced future eating disorder onset in certain subsets of the participants included in trials (eg, at 1 of the 2 sites included in one large efficacy trial).[47] Student Bodies is a cognitive-behavior Internet-based program, wherein participants journal and engage in group discussion supervised by a clinician, and it includes content aimed at reducing weight and shape concerns, informing participants about the risks associated with eating disorders and how to engage in healthy living practices, for 8 weeks. Jones and colleagues[48] recruited high school students who were at or above the 85th percentile BMI for their age and who reported having at least 1 binge episode per week for the past 3 months to receive either a modified, 16-week version of Student Bodies focusing on weight stabilization and healthy living practices or to a waitlist control, making this 1 of the only indicated prevention programs to be evaluated. Student Bodies participants showed a significant reduction in binge episodes and BMI compared with the waitlist control group. A majority of participants in the Student Bodies condition, however, completed only 7 or fewer weeks of the 16-week intervention, raising concerns about acceptability. Student Bodies has not been evaluated by independent research teams or evaluated in effectiveness trials.

Student Athlete Eating Disorder Prevention Program

An intervention designed to prevent the onset of eating disorders in adolescent female and male elite athletes prevented the future onset of eating disorders and reduced symptoms associated with eating disorders in adolescent female athletes over a 1-year follow-up relative to assessment-only controls.[49] In this school-based group intervention, adolescent male and female high school athletes seek to improve self-esteem through self-efficacy and learn the meaning of intrinsic versus extrinsic motivation and mastery versus performance goals to emphasize the importance of deriving strength from oneself rather than performance issues and significant others. The program was efficacious in preventing eating disorders in female athletes and reduced symptoms associated with eating disorders but had limited effects on male athletes. This prevention program has not been evaluated by independent research teams or in effectiveness trials.

Mindfulness Eating Disorder Prevention

In 1 randomized control trial, women ages 17 to 31 who reported body image concerns but did not have an eating disorder were randomly assigned to a mindfulness-based intervention (MBI), a dissonance-based intervention loosely based on the Body Project, or an assessment-only control.[50] In the MBI, participants practiced mindfulness, discussed barriers to engaging in mindfulness, and completed exercises aimed at countering negative body image–related thoughts both in group sessions and as homework, which should help participants more effectively counter and experience less negative affect from these thoughts in future situations.[50] The MBI produced significant reductions in eating disorder symptoms relative to the assessment-only controls at the postintervention assessment, but these effects did not persist over longer-term follow-up. MBI has not been evaluated in any additional trials by this research team or other teams and it has not been evaluated in effectiveness trials.

SUMMARY AND DIRECTIONS FOR FUTURE RESEARCH

In summary, 4 eating disorder prevention programs have been found to reduce eating disorder onset and/or eating disorder symptoms. In addition, the evidence base for eating disorder prevention programs often includes rigorous tests of the intervention theory and effectiveness trials that determine whether the program works under ecologically valid conditions. There are several important directions for future research. First, it will be critical to determine how to improve the efficacy of existing evidence-based eating disorder prevention programs. Second, it would be useful to examine factors that influence adoption and implementation of evidence-based eating disorder prevention programs as well as factors that predict fidelity, competence, and sustainability of intervention delivery. Third, emerging evidence suggests that pursuit of the thin beauty ideal, body dissatisfaction, and reported dieting predict future onset of bulimia nervosa, binge-eating disorder, and purging disorder but not future onset of anorexia nervosa. Because most prevention programs target individuals with body dissatisfaction and attempt to reduce pursuit of the thin beauty ideal, body dissatisfaction, and unhealthy weight control behaviors, this implies that existing prevention programs may be ineffective in preventing restricting anorexia nervosa. It will be important for trials to evaluate whether evidence-based eating disorder prevention programs actually reduce onset of all types of eating disorders. Fourth, it will be vital to continue to conduct prospective risk factor studies to advance knowledge of subgroups at elevated risk for eating disorder onset and additional risk factors, including biological factors that predict future onset of eating disorders, because this information should inform the design of even more effective prevention programs. There is a particular need to conduct prospective studies to elucidate risk factors that predict future onset of eating disorders in boys and men and to translate these findings into effective prevention programs for boys and men.

REFERENCES

1. Dakanalis A, Clerici M, Bartoli F, et al. Risk and maintenance factors for young women's DSM-5 eating disorders. Arch Womens Ment Health 2017;20(6):721–31.
2. Swanson S, Crow S, Le Grange D, et al. Prevalence and correlates of eating disorders in adolescents: results from the national comorbidity survey replication adolescent supplement. Arch Gen Psychiatry 2011;68(7):714–23.
3. Stice E, Bohon C. Eating disorders. In: Beauchaine TP, Hinshaw SP, editors. Child and adolescent psychopathology. Hoboken (NJ): Wiley and Sons; 2013. p. 715–38.
4. Stice E, Gau JM, Rohde P, et al. Risk factors that predict future onset of each DSM-5 eating disorder: predictive specificity in high-risk adolescent females. J Abnorm Psychol 2017;126(1):38–51.
5. Cnattingius S, Hultman CM, Dahl M, et al. Very preterm birth, birth trauma, and the risk of anorexia nervosa among girls. Arch Gen Psychiatry 1999;56(7):634.
6. Kotler L, Cohen P, Davies M, et al. Longitudinal relationships between childhood, adolescent, and adult eating disorders. J Am Acad Child Adolesc Psychiatry 2001;40(12):1434–40.
7. Tyrka AR, Waldron I, Graber JA, et al. Prospective predictors of the onset of anorexic and bulimic syndromes. Int J Eat Disord 2002;32(3):282–90.
8. Patton GC, Johnson-Sabine E, Wood K, et al. Abnormal eating attitudes in London schoolgirls — a prospective epidemiological study: outcome at twelve month follow-up. Psychol Med 1990;20(02):383.
9. Killen J, Taylor C, Hayward C, et al. Weight concerns influence the development of eating disorders: a 4-year prospective study. J Consult Clin Psychol 1996; 64(5):936–40. Available at: http://psycnet.apa.org/buy/1996-00478-014. Accessed July 3, 2018.
10. Patton GC, Selzer R, Coffey C, et al. Onset of adolescent eating disorders: population based cohort study over 3 years. BMJ 1999;318(7186):765–8.
11. Stice E, Davis K, Miller NP, et al. Fasting increases risk for onset of binge eating and bulimic pathology: a 5-year prospective study. J Abnorm Psychol 2008; 117(4):941–6.
12. Stice E, Marti CN, Durant S. Risk factors for onset of eating disorders: Evidence of multiple risk pathways from an 8-year prospective study. Behav Res Ther 2011; 49(10):622–7.
13. Santonastaso P, Friederici S, Favaro A. Full and partial syndromes in eating disorders: a 1-year prospective study of risk factors among female students. Psychopathology 1999;32(1):50–6.
14. Ghaderi A, Scott B. Prevalence, incidence and prospective risk factors for eating disorders. Acta Psychiatr Scand 2001;104(2):122–30.
15. The McKnight Investigators TM. Risk factors for the onset of eating disorders in adolescent girls: results of the mcknight longitudinal risk factor study. Am J Psychiatry 2003;160(2):248–54.
16. Jacobi C, Fittig E, Bryson SW, et al. Who is really at risk? Identifying risk factors for subthreshold and full syndrome eating disorders in a high-risk sample. Psychol Med 2011;41(9):1939–49.

17. Rohde P, Stice E, Marti CN. Development and predictive effects of eating disorder risk factors during adolescence: Implications for prevention efforts. Int J Eat Disord 2015;48(2):187–98.
18. Johnson JG, Cohen P, Kasen S, et al. Childhood adversities associated with risk for eating disorders or weight problems during adolescence or early adulthood. Am J Psychiatry 2002. https://doi.org/10.1176/APPI.AJP.159.3.394.
19. Martínez-González MA, Gual P, Lahortiga F, et al. Parental factors, mass media influences, and the onset of eating disorders in a prospective population-based cohort. Pediatrics 2003;111(2):315–20.
20. Beato-Fernandez L, Rodriguez-Cano T, Belmonte-Llario A, et al. Risk factors for eating disorders in adolescents. Eur Child Adolesc Psychiatry 2004;13(5): 287–94.
21. Allen KL, Byrne SM, Forbes D, et al. Risk factors for full- and partial-syndrome early adolescent eating disorders: a population-based pregnancy cohort study. J Am Acad Child Adolesc Psychiatry 2009;48(8):800–9.
22. Allen KL, Byrne SM, Oddy WH, et al. Risk factors for binge eating and purging eating disorders: differences based on age of onset. Int J Eat Disord 2014; 47(7):802–12.
23. Stice E, Marti CN, Spoor S, et al. Dissonance and healthy weight eating disorder prevention programs: Long-term effects from a randomized efficacy trial. J Consult Clin Psychol 2008;76(2):329–40.
24. Stice E, Shaw H, Burton E, et al. Dissonance and healthy weight eating disorder prevention programs: a randomized efficacy trial. J Consult Clin Psychol 2006; 74(2):263–75.
25. Festinger L. A theory of cognitive dissonance. Stanford (CA): Stanford University Press; 1957.
26. Brown T, Keel P. A randomized controlled trial of a peer co-led dissonance-based eating disorder prevention program for gay men. Behav Res Ther 2015;74:1–10.
27. Rohde P, Stice E, Shaw H, et al. Age effects in eating disorder baseline risk factors and prevention intervention effects. Int J Eat Disord 2017;50(11):1273–80.
28. Rodriguez R, Marchand E, Ng J, et al. Effects of a cognitive-dissonance-based eating disorder prevention program are similar for Asian American, Hispanic, and White participants. Int J Eat Disord 2008;41(7):618–25.
29. Stice E, Marti C, Cheng Z. Effectiveness of a dissonance-based eating disorder prevention program for ethnic groups in two randomized controlled trials. Behav Res Ther 2014;55:54–64.
30. Becker C, Smith L, Ciao A. Reducing eating disorder risk factors in sorority members: a randomized trial. Behav Ther 2005;36:245–53. Available at: https://digitalcommons.trinity.edu/psych_faculty/6. Accessed July 3, 2018.
31. Halliwell E, Diedrichs PC. Testing a dissonance body image intervention among young girls. Health Psychol 2014;33(2):201–4.
32. Mitchell KS, Mazzeo SE, Rausch SM, et al. Innovative interventions for disordered eating: Evaluating dissonance-based and yoga interventions. Int J Eat Disord 2007;40(2):120–8.
33. Serdar K, Kelly NR, Palmberg AA, et al. Comparing online and face-to-face dissonance-based eating disorder prevention. Eat Disord 2014;22(3):244–60.
34. Green M, Scott N, Diyankova I, et al. Eating disorder prevention: an experimental comparison of high level dissonance, low level dissonance, and no-treatment control. Eat Disord 2005;13(2):157–69.

35. McMillan W, Stice E, Rohde P. High- and low-level dissonance-based eating disorder prevention programs with young women with body image concerns: An experimental trial. J Consult Clin Psychol 2011;79(1):129–34.
36. Stice E, Yokum S, Waters A. Dissonance-based eating disorder prevention program reduces reward region response to thin models; how actions shape valuation. PLoS One 2015;10(12):e0144530.
37. Stice E, Rohde P, Butryn ML, et al. Effectiveness trial of a selective dissonance-based eating disorder prevention program with female college students: Effects at 2- and 3-year follow-up. Behav Res Ther 2015;71:20–6.
38. Stice E, Rohde P, Shaw H, et al. An effectiveness trial of a selected dissonance-based eating disorder prevention program for female high school students: Long-term effects. J Consult Clin Psychol 2011;79(4):500–8.
39. Becker CB, McDaniel L, Bull S, et al. Can we reduce eating disorder risk factors in female college athletes? A randomized exploratory investigation of two peer-led interventions. Body Image 2012;9(1):31–42.
40. Ciao AC, Latner JD, Brown KE, et al. Effectiveness of a peer-delivered dissonance-based program in reducing eating disorder risk factors in high school girls. Int J Eat Disord 2015;48(6):779–84.
41. Halliwell E, Jarman H, McNamara A, et al. Dissemination of evidence-based body image interventions: a pilot study into the effectiveness of using undergraduate students as interventionists in secondary schools. Body Image 2015;14:1–4.
42. Stice E, Rohde P, Durant S, et al. Effectiveness of peer-led dissonance-based eating disorder prevention groups: Results from two randomized pilot trials. Behav Res Ther 2013;51(4–5):197–206.
43. Stice E, Rohde P, Shaw H, et al. Clinician-led, peer-led, and Internet-delivered dissonance-based eating disorder prevention programs: acute effectiveness of these delivery modalities. J Consult Clin Psychol 2017;85(9):883–9.
44. Stice E, Rohde P, Shaw H, et al. Efficacy trial of a selective prevention program targeting both eating disorder symptoms and unhealthy weight gain among female college students. J Consult Clin Psychol 2012;80(1):164–70.
45. Stice E, Rohde P, Shaw H, et al. Efficacy trial of a selective prevention program targeting both eating disorders and obesity among female college students: 1- and 2-year follow-up effects. J Consult Clin Psychol 2013;81(1):183–9.
46. Stice E, Yokum S, Burger K, et al. Physiology & Behavior A pilot randomized trial of a cognitive reappraisal obesity prevention program 2017. Physiol Behav 2015;138:124–32.
47. Taylor CB, Bryson S, Luce KH, et al. Prevention of eating disorders in at-risk college-age women. Arch Gen Psychiatry 2006;63(8):881.
48. Jones M, Luce K, Osborne K, et al. Randomized, controlled trial of an internet-facilitated intervention for reducing binge eating and overweight in adolescents. Pediatrics 2008;121(3):453–62.
49. Martinsen M, Bahr R, Borresen R, et al. Preventing eating disorders among young elite athletes: a randomized controlled trial. Med Sci Sports Exerc 2014;46(3):435–47.
50. Atkinson MJ, Wade TD. Does mindfulness have potential in eating disorders prevention? A preliminary controlled trial with young adult women. Early Interv Psychiatry 2016;10(3):234–45.

The Second Wave of Public Policy Advocacy for Eating Disorders

Charting the Course to Maximize Population Impact

S. Bryn Austin, ScD[a,b,c,d],*, Rebecca Hutcheson, MSW[d,e], Shalini Wickramatilake-Templeman, MHS[d,1], Katrina Velasquez, Esq, MA[f,2]

KEYWORDS

• Eating disorders • Policy • Advocacy • Mental health • Prevention • Early detection
• Treatment • Recovery

KEY POINTS

• Eating disorders research funding is significantly less than that allotted to other serious illnesses, especially when considering the numbers affected and the disability-adjusted life years lost.

• The first wave of US public policy advocacy for eating disorders has shown promise, with passage of federal 21st Century Cures Act in 2016 as a crowning achievement.

• To maximize the impact of primary, secondary, tertiary prevention of eating disorders, a second wave of policy advocacy is needed to target the structural determinants of eating disorders and remedy the inequities in underfunding and inadequate focus on these serious illnesses.

• For ethical and pragmatic reasons, mental health clinicians and researchers should engage in public policy advocacy for eating disorders.

• Collaborative governance initiatives are among the most promising approaches to maximize impact to improve outcomes and reduce the societal burden of eating disorders.

Disclosure Statement: K. Velasquez is a consultant for the Residential Eating Disorders Consortium, a nonprofit trade association for eating disorders treatment centers.

[a] Department of Social and Behavioral Sciences, Harvard T.H. Chan School of Public Health, Boston, MA, USA; [b] Department of Pediatrics, Harvard Medical School, Boston, MA, USA; [c] Division of Adolescent and Young Adult Medicine, Boston Children's Hospital, 333 Longwood Avenue, Room 634, Boston, MA 02115, USA; [d] Strategic Training Initiative for the Prevention of Eating Disorders: A Public Health Incubator, Boston, MA, USA; [e] Department of Health Services, University of Washington School of Public Health, Health and Public Health Systems Research, The University of Washington, 1959 Northeast Pacific Street, Box 357660, Seattle, WA 98195, USA; [f] Center Road Solutions, LLC, Washington, DC, USA

[1] Present address: 1919 Pennsylvania Avenue, Northwest, Suite M-250, Washington, DC 20006.
[2] Present address: 1140 3rd Street, Northeast, 2nd Floor, Washington, DC 20002.
* Corresponding author. Division of Adolescent and Young Adult Medicine, Boston Children's Hospital, 333 Longwood Avenue, Room 634, Boston, MA 02115.
E-mail address: bryn.austin@childrens.harvard.edu

Psychiatr Clin N Am 42 (2019) 319–336
https://doi.org/10.1016/j.psc.2019.01.013
0193-953X/19/© 2019 Elsevier Inc. All rights reserved.

Abbreviations	
CDC	Centers for Disease Control and Prevention
CMHS	Center for Mental Health Services
HHS	Department of Health and Human Services
NIMH	National Institutes of Mental Health
SAMHSA	Substance Use and Mental Health Services Administration

INTRODUCTION

In late 2018, the Lancet Commission on Global Mental Health published a report warning of the threat that the global mental health crisis poses to sustainable economic development and human rights around the world.[1] Globally, mental health and substance use disorders are the leading cause of years lived with disability.[2] The Commission's comprehensive and far-reaching report also issued a call for profound changes in national responses to the crises, asserting that more than 13 million deaths globally each year could be prevented and an estimated US$16 trillion saved by 2030 if appropriate mental health services were made available worldwide.[1,3] The report paints a stark picture of inadequacy of government mental health programs and services, not only in low-income and emerging economies, but also in high-income countries, including the United States.[1]

The response to our nation's mental health crisis broadly and eating disorders specifically has fallen short of objectives. The World Health Organization estimates less than 20% of Americans with anxiety, mood, or substance use disorders have accessed mental health services in the prior 12 months.[4] One study examining the amount of US National Institutes of Health research funding for 29 common health conditions as a function of condition-specific disability-adjusted life-years lost found that depression, among the most prevalent of mental illnesses, received substantially less funding than all other illnesses evaluated, most of which were physical health conditions.[5]

Deficits in the United States' response to eating disorders are even more notably pronounced. An estimated 30 million Americans are affected by an eating disorder in their lifetime and millions more are affected by subclinical disorders that are debilitating and sometimes deadly.[6–8] Eating disorders arguably have the highest mortality of any psychiatric disorder,[9,10] and an adolescent with anorexia nervosa has nearly 10 times the risk of dying than a same age healthy peer.[11] Effective treatments for a range of eating disorders are well-established,[9,12,13] and yet the vast majority of those affected never access treatment.[6,14,15] Furthermore, there are notable deficits in early detection: it is well-documented that symptoms are routinely missed in males, communities of color, and higher weight individuals with eating disorders.[15–18] Additionally, federal research funding for eating disorders amounts to a small fraction of funding allotted to other serious illnesses, especially when taking into account the illness burden on individuals, their families, and society. For instance, in 2017, the National Institutes of Health funded research for Alzheimer's disease at approximately $239 per affected individual, autism at $109, and schizophrenia at $69, whereas, for eating disorders research, the National Institutes of Health awarded approximately $1 per affected individual.[19] Furthermore, in an examination of the National Institutes of Mental Health (NIMH) research funding for 7 major mental health conditions relative to disability-adjusted life-years lost as a consequence of each condition, 2013 research funding for eating disorders was the most disproportionately underfunded compared with all other conditions included.[20]

RECOMMENDATIONS FROM THE *LANCET* COMMISSION ON GLOBAL MENTAL HEALTH

The significant gaps in the United States' response to mental illness generally and eating disorders specifically are daunting, but much work has been done to identify productive lines of inquiry and intervention to move toward meaningful solutions. To start, we can turn to the *Lancet* Commission report, which offers a set of recommended actions for the global community that are applicable to addressing gaps in eating disorders treatment and research in the United States:[1]

1. Integrate mental health services: Scale up and fully integrate mental health services into primary care and other medical specialties to address the constraints on the availability of care and ensure adequate coverage for treatment.
2. Reduce mental health stigma and lack of awareness: Mitigate the many barriers to care and threats to mental health, such as a lack of understanding of and attention to the importance of mental health promotion and the consequences of mental illness across sectors, widespread stigma and discrimination related to mental health that substantially inhibits people from obtaining needed services, and growing inequalities in access to resources, particularly for lower socioeconomic populations.
3. Initiate intersectoral collaborations for policy change: Initiate public policies and community development through intersectoral collaborations involving government, mental health experts and advocates with personal mental illness experience, and stakeholders from a wide range of nonhealth arenas, such as education, workplaces, criminal justice, and other fields.
4. Innovate with technologic and nonspecialist delivery: Prioritize innovations in telemental health, digital technologies, and trained nonspecialists (ie, community lay health workers) to develop and evaluate new treatment modalities to vastly expand access to mental health support and treatment.
5. Enhance primary and secondary prevention through new investments and established platforms: Augment resource investment in mental health training and services by investing new funds and harnessing existing funding for related and compatible efforts within established platforms and increase funding for interventions for mental health promotion as primary prevention and early intervention (secondary prevention) for incipient mental distress.
6. Fund transdisciplinary research for primary, secondary, and tertiary prevention: Increase funding for transdisciplinary research for elucidation of underlying causes and mechanisms of mental disorder to inform primary (ie, intervention before onset of symptoms), secondary (ie, early detection of incipient disease), and tertiary (ie, treatment to shorten course, ameliorate sequelae of disease, and improve survival) preventive interventions.[21]

The *Lancet* Commission recommendations are aspirational, setting stretch goals far beyond what currently exists in global mental health care delivery. Although these recommendations did not specifically address eating disorders, the recommendations can serve as a template, developed through consensus of global mental health experts, to measure the degree to which US public policy advocacy for eating disorders is appropriately targeted and where efforts need to be strengthened.

THE FIRST WAVE OF EATING DISORDERS PUBLIC POLICY ADVOCACY: MANY SUCCESSES, MUCH WORK STILL TO BE DONE

Over the last decade and particularly in the past 5 years, the community has made progress in advancing eating disorder-specific federal and state public policy initiatives, all of which align with one or another of the *Lancet* Commission recommendations. In this article, we focus specifically on public policy advocacy to refer to efforts to influence laws, government regulations, guidance, and funding programs promulgated through the legislative and administrative branches of the US government.[22] Although advocacy through the judicial branch of government, such as class action suits to compel insurers to conform to the Paul Wellstone and Pete Domenici Mental Health Parity and Addiction Equity Act of 2008 (Public Law 110–343), is also a powerful lever for change for the eating disorders community, that aspect of advocacy is beyond the scope of this article.

For example, pertinent to *Lancet* Commission recommendation 1 to integrate mental health services into health insurance coverage and into primary and other medical care systems, the eating disorders community was actively involved in securing the passage of the federal mental health parity, which was intended to require that group health plans and health insurers provide mental health and substance use disorder benefits commensurate with medical/surgical coverage. Disappointment with the implementation of this law and the gaps created by the final rule that delegated authority to states for delineating mental health conditions covered as essential health benefits and expanded the Mental Health Parity and Addiction Equity Act of 2008 to individual and small group plans under the Patient Protection and Affordable Care Act then motivated the eating disorders community's similarly active engagement in securing the passage in 2016 of the 21st Century Cures Act (Public Law 114–255), which was the first US federal law in history to specifically address eating disorders. This legislative success was the crowning achievement of the first wave of US eating disorders public policy advocacy. The law included provisions clarifying that eating disorders are a mental illness and, when covered by insurance, must be covered without discrimination for levels of care and subdisorder. The federal Department of Labor has now issued guidance on how insurance plans should cover eating disorders treatment.

Additionally, the eating disorders community has secured several state policy advocacy successes. For instance, Missouri expanded parity with a law passed in 2015 that specifically requires eating disorders coverage by health insurers in addition to a requirement that, if an individual does not have insurance coverage or financial assistance for diagnosis or treatment, the Department of Health and Senior Services must provide assistance and coverage. A number of critical state laws were passed in 2017 and 2018 related to eating disorders insurance coverage, increasing access to care, and licensure of eating disorders treatment centers in Illinois, Maine, Missouri, Montana, Washington, and West Virginia. Unfortunately, in 2017 and 2018 West Virginia and Montana passed laws to limit eating disorders insurance coverage under mental health parity to persons diagnosed with anorexia nervosa and bulimia nervosa, excluding those with other eating disorders such as binge eating disorder and serious subclinical eating disorder syndromes.

Relevant to *Lancet* Commission recommendation 2 to decrease mental health stigma and increase awareness, the federal 21st Century Cures Act requires that the US Department of Health and Human Services (HHS) Office on Women's Health provide accurate and evidence-based information on eating disorders to the public. Also, the US Senate passed a National Eating Disorders Awareness Week resolution in 2018, and various state and jurisdictions (Alabama, California, Connecticut, New Jersey, and Puerto Rico) passed similar awareness resolutions in 2017 and 2018. Missouri passed into law in 2010 a requirement that state programs include eating disorders awareness and education, which should be done in collaboration with departments overseeing health, senior services, and education as well as any additional state department as the Department of Mental Health sees fit. With a law focused specifically on the fashion industry, California passed a law in 2018 mandating that talent agencies provide education on eating disorders, their risks, and healthy nutrition to fashion models working in the state. Unfortunately, several federal and state policies persist that contribute to weight stigma and eating disorders, especially those that restrict access to insurance coverage for employees at higher weights and require school-based body mass index screening among children and youth regardless of risk for eating disorders.

Aligned with *Lancet* Commission recommendation 5 to enhance primary and secondary prevention through both new funding and established platforms, the 21st Century Cures Act included provisions that HHS provide training for health care professionals in the primary, secondary, and tertiary prevention of eating disorders. As a result, in 2018 the federal Substance Use and Mental Health Services Administration (SAMHSA) awarded a $3.75 million, 5-year grant for the first Center of Excellence for Eating Disorders to provide this training to providers nationwide. In addition, an interagency working group, including a number of HHS offices and agencies (Office on Women's Health, SAMHSA, NIMH, Health Resources Services Administration, Agency for Health Care Quality and Research, Centers for Disease Control and Prevention [CDC], and US Food and Drug Administration), collaborated with community partners to offer the federal government's first online training for pediatric primary care providers in the early detection of eating disorders. As a result of strong advocacy, in both the 2018 and 2019 federal budget bills, Congress passed provisions urging the Health Resources Services Administration to integrate eating disorders early identification training for health care professionals within the agency's $49 million Primary Care Training and Enhancement grant program. Congress passed language within the Fiscal Year 2019 Department of Defense and Labor, HHS, and Education Appropriations Act, 2019 (Public Law 115–245) urging surveillance of eating disorders signs and symptoms in youth within the CDC's Youth Risk Behavioral Surveillance System, which—if these data were to be collected—would allow states to assess some indicators of burden of illness of eating disorders and evaluate the effectiveness of any policy initiatives to promote prevention.

Finally, pertinent to *Lancet* Commission recommendation 6 to fund transdisciplinary research for primary, secondary, and tertiary prevention, the NIMH, from 2009 to 2013, awarded on average approximately $15 million per year to eating disorders-related research,[20] although mostly focused on treatment and genetics and not necessarily for transdisciplinary research. Congress recently invested in eating disorders research funding for military members, veterans, and their families by including eating disorders as a topic area for research funding within the Department of Defense's Peer-Reviewed Medical Research Program for 2017 through 2019 federal fiscal years, providing approximately $5 million in eating disorders research funding per year.

The achievements of the eating disorders community's first wave of US public policy advocacy, with the passage of the 21st Century Cures Act in 2016, are encouraging and a testament to the importance of a coordinated strategy of multiple community stakeholders to effect policy change. Notably absent are advocacy victories aligned with *Lancet* Commission recommendations 3 and 4. Despite substantial first wave victories, we are left with the reality that, compared with other mental health conditions and medical conditions, the nation's response to serious eating disorders is grossly inadequate to reduce the burden of illness or meet existing needs. We must continue to chart a course for the future of public policy advocacy for eating disorders, a course that sets a new, higher standard for a more comprehensive approach with even greater impact than that achieved in the first wave.

A STRATEGIC PLAN FOR THE SECOND WAVE
Second-Wave Strategy 1: Leverage Existing Government Platforms

The next wave of advocacy should begin with a systematic assessment of a wide range of government agencies and offices at the federal, state, and local levels to identify established relevant platforms that could be extended to include attention to eating disorders primary, secondary, and tertiary prevention. On a federal level, the Medicaid Early and Periodic Screening, Diagnosis, and Treatment program requires providers to assess symptoms of mental health concerns in children and adolescents; therefore, working within this existing structure, Medicaid could create guidance to clarify that eating disorders should also be assessed. In another federal-level example, the following case study highlights established platforms and activities within SAMHSA that could be adapted to expand and deepen the agency's response to the eating disorders crisis.

Case example: second-wave policy advocacy recommendations focused on the Substance Abuse and Mental Health Services Administration recommendations

Recommendation a: Ensure that SAMHSA includes eating disorders in its efforts to address serious mental illness.

SAMHSA should be one of the leading federal agencies for focus of eating disorder public policy advocacy, because its mandate is to address mental health and substance use disorders in all its programs and policies. Beyond the newly funded Center of Excellence for Eating Disorders mentioned elsewhere in this article, SAMHSA has the potential to advance the primary, secondary, and tertiary prevention of eating disorders. SAMHSA has various offices and centers that provide national leadership and assistance for quality mental health and substance use disorder services while supporting states, territories, tribes, communities, and local organizations through grants and contract awards. One of SAMHSA's centers, the Center for Mental Health Services (CMHS), leads federal efforts to promote the prevention and treatment of mental disorders. Congress created CMHS to bring hope for a better quality of life to adults who have a serious mental illness and children with emotional disorders. Specifically, the role of CMHS is to[23]:

- Strengthen the nation's mental health system by helping states improve and increase the quality and range of their treatment, rehabilitation, and support;
- Make it easier for people to access mental health programs;
- Encourage a range of programs, such as systems of care, to respond to the increasing number of mental, emotional, and behavioral problems among the nation's children;
- Support outreach and case management programs for the thousands of Americans who are homeless and foster improvement of these services; and
- Ensure that scientifically established findings and practice-based knowledge are applied in preventing and treating mental disorders.

The NIMH defines a serious mental illness as "a mental, behavioral, or emotional disorder resulting in serious functional impairment, which substantially interferes with or limits one or more major life activities."[24] As a serious mental illness, eating disorders should be characterized by SAMHSA as such in all of its materials and programs, which will help to underscore their appropriate place within the agency's mandate and open up many funding opportunities for the eating disorders field in the long-term within existing platforms already developed by SAMHSA and funded by Congress.

Recommendation b: Authorize and fund a grant program to be administered by SAMHSA to increase access to eating disorders treatment services.

Considering that eating disorders are among the most serious of mental illnesses that can greatly inhibit functioning and undermine quality of life, SAMHSA/CMHS should administer a grant program to provide treatment services to individuals who are otherwise unable to access appropriate services owing to a lack of insurance coverage. This type of program would follow the model of existing programs CMHS already offer for other serious mental illness and substance use disorders and could be organized within existing structures. For instance, as is currently done with other conditions, grants could fund established state mental health program directors (who would then contract with providers in their state) or could be administered directly to providers. If grants were to go to state mental health program directors, there would likely need to be further eating disorders advocacy efforts within states to ensure some funding is allocated to eating disorders providers in competitive grants. This would also encourage mental health providers to be involved in federal advocacy efforts to ensure passage of any grant authorization bill and subsequent implementation.

Recommendation c: HHS through the Assistant Secretary for Mental Health and Substance Use should lead cross-agency and cross-departmental work on eating disorders.

As a leading agency within the federal government on mental health issues, SAMHSA should coordinate with any other HHS agencies and departments that are currently or should be actively involved in eating disorders-related work (eg, CDC, Health Resources Services Administration, US Food and Drug Administration, Indian Health Services, Federal Trade Commission, Agency for International Development, Departments of Agriculture, Justice, Commerce, Education, Labor, Defense) to ensure that efforts are complementary and not duplicative, and to ensure that opportunities to integrate innovations for the primary, secondary, and tertiary prevention of eating disorders are identified and pursued. A cross-agency and cross-departmental committee led by HHS through the Assistant Secretary for Mental Health and Substance Use would elevate eating disorders concerns at the federal level and keep attention focused and sustained. An existing example of this type of collaborative coordinating work is the Interdepartmental Serious Mental Illness Coordinating Committee. Any federal coordinating committee focused on eating disorders must include those personally affected by eating disorders, researchers, clinicians, and stakeholders with a wide range of expertise pertinent to primary, secondary, and tertiary prevention.

Second-Wave Strategy 2: Develop Policy Initiatives Targeting Structural Determinants of Poor Health and Health Inequities

The Lancet Commission recommendations serve as a useful reference to assess the pertinence of advocacy targets, based on global expert consensus, but they do not gauge the potential impact of one target versus another and thus prioritize advocacy efforts. To evaluate one proposed target for policy advocacy versus another, we can use a framework developed nearly a decade ago by former CDC director Thomas Frieden.[25] Frieden proposed the Health Impact Pyramid to delineate a hierarchy of relative potential for the large-scale, population impact of different approaches to health disparities and the major causes of illness, disability, and death (**Fig. 1**). Drawing on decades of empirical data on the public health impact of different intervention strategies, Frieden's central thesis was that the types of interventions that target individuals for change in behavior or for clinical treatment of existing

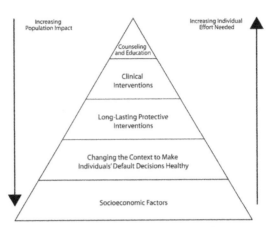

Increasing
Population Impact

Increasing Individual
Effort Needed

Counseling
and Education

Clinical
Interventions

Long-Lasting Protective
Interventions

Changing the Context to Make
Individuals' Default Decisions Healthy

Socioeconomic Factors

Fig. 1. Health impact pyramid depicting hierarchy of potential impact on population health by intervention type and target. (*From* Frieden TR. A framework for public health action: the health impact pyramid. Am J Public Health 2010;100(4):591; with permission.)

disease—especially the top 2 tiers of the 5-tier pyramid—are comparatively the easiest to develop and deliver in our current public health and health care infrastructure and consequently receive the most attention, but also are the least impactful because they do not change the conditions that produce illness in the first place. A focus on individually targeted behavior change and educational interventions, he succinctly writes, "is symptomatic of failure to establish contexts in which healthy choices are default actions."[25] Similarly, a focus on refining evidence-based care to be received by the small portion of the population that will have access to it—as is the case in the US health care system, where there is no guarantee of health coverage or access to any kind of mental health or specifically eating disorders care in many areas of the country and for many in marginalized communities[6,15,26,27]—is destined to ultimately be of only moderate impact on the population as a whole. With this reasoning, Frieden urged us to expand our attention especially to include the lower 2 tiers of the pyramid that target social and structural determinants of health, where the potential for large-scale population impact is greatest.[25] The decades of research documenting a range of social and structural determinants of the health and mental health inequities—such as vastly unequal distribution of economic resources and discrimination in law and criminal justice—make clear why public policy interventions must target those determinants to effectively reduce and eliminate inequities.[28,29] However, Frieden also noted, as have many other health policy advocacy and social justice scholars,[1,22,30] that changing the conditions that produce and perpetuate illness—that is, working within the lower tiers of the Health Impact Pyramid rather than exclusively in the upper tiers of the pyramid—requires significantly more effort, planning, collaboration, and political will. This is where intersectoral partnerships become most essential, as proposed by the *Lancet* Commission (recommendation 3) and others.[30]

In **Table 1**, the authors provide target recommendations for second-wave public policy advocacy in eating disorders. To help illuminate both the target and potential impact of our recommendations, we categorize each recommendation according to its pertinence to both the 6 *Lancet* Commission recommendations (1–6) described herein and the 5 tiers of the Health Impact Pyramid depicted in **Fig. 1**. Whereas the first wave of eating disorders public policy advocacy primarily addressed the upper

Table 1
Example public policy recommendations for second-wave advocacy for primary, secondary, and tertiary prevention of ED, categorized according to Frieden health impact pyramid tiers and *Lancet* report recommendations

Tiers of Health Impact Pyramid[25]	Examples of Public Policy Recommendations
Individually targeted counseling, education for behavior change	Mandate mental health, nutrition, and/or health education that addresses weight and shape control behavior and body image counseling in school systems. *(LC1)*[a]
	Require that behaviorally targeted nutrition and physical activity studies and programs funded by government through NIH and other health/mental health research programs include evaluation of unintended exacerbating effects on weight stigma and disordered eating and protocols to protect against such negative effects of the research. *(LC5)*
	Require that behaviorally targeted nutrition and physical activity programs funded by government through the HHS, Education, Justice, etc, and similar state-, county-, or city-funded program include protocols to protect against unintended exacerbating effects on weight stigma and disordered eating. *(LC5)*
Individually targeted medical, psychiatric interventions	Ensure that SAMHSA and other federal agencies classify ED as "serious mental illness" so that regulation stipulating procedures and funding addressing serious mental illness include ED. *(LC1)*
	Ensure that Medicare, Medicaid, Indian Health Services, Department of Defense's TRICARE for military members and their families, and Veterans Administration's VA-CHAMPS require comprehensive ED treatment coverage for their beneficiaries. *(LC1)*
	Ensure that the CMS require ED screening be included in Medicaid mandated EPSDT program and, if the PHQ-9 used, require follow up if item #5 on dysregulation of eating behavior endorsed. *(LC1)*
	Require inclusion of ED in HRSA SBIRT program to evaluate the potential use of an SBIRT approach for ED. *(LC1, LC5)*
	Mandate that HRSA require Federally Qualified Health Centers adopt routine screening for ED in primary care and offer referrals to effective treatment. *(LC1, LC5)*
	Require HHS and/or appropriate state-level administrators include ED in planning, service delivery, data collection, and data reporting requirements for recipients of community mental health block grant funds. *(LC1, LC6)*
	Require federal agencies to fund pilot projects to address ED within their respective flexible funding mechanisms (eg, HRSA Special Projects of National Significance) and to include ED in agency-supported training programs (such as HRSA Maternal and Child Health Bureau Leadership Education in Adolescent Health programs). *(LC1)*
	HHS should fund and coordinate the training of health care providers in the ED early detection (secondary prevention) and treatment (tertiary prevention) through Centers of Excellence for Eating Disorders and through other provider training programs administered by other HHS agencies and other federal programs. Federal programs should offer webinars and other trainings with continuing education credits for recipients of federal funding. *(LC1, LC5)*

(continued on next page)

Table 1
(continued)

Tiers of Health Impact Pyramid[25]	Examples of Public Policy Recommendations
	Similar ED training of health care providers should be pursued on the state, county, and city levels, such as through the National Association of State Mental Health Program Directors and National Association of County and City Health officials. *(LC1, LC5)*
	HRSA should fund and coordinate training of community lay health nonspecialists to provide primary, secondary, and tertiary prevention of ED. *(LC4)*
	Ensure all psychiatric diagnoses in the DSM-5 are covered by federal and state mental health parity laws; create parity regulations when absent, such as within Indian Health Services; enhance enforcement of mental health parity laws at state and federal levels and for military personnel and dependents.
	Department of Labor and state insurance commissioners should require that mental health professionals be involved in reviewing health insurance claims; streamline ED insurance claim processes; enforce mental health parity for employer-based insurance plans; and require insurance plan coverage for ED treatment. *(LC1)*
	Ensure ED treatment covered in all health plans, including short-term health plans and Association Health Plans. *(LC1).*
	CMS should require programs using technology innovations and tele-mental health funded by government to include ED treatment. *(LC4)*
	Ensure ED screening and treatment is offered through any mental health and substance use treatment programs led or funded by government at the federal, state, county, or city level. *(LC1, LC5)*
Long-lasting, individually targeted protective interventions (ie, resiliency, "inoculation")	Fund research into development, evaluation, and implementation of effective socioemotional health promotion and skills training interventions that include attention to ED risk factors through the CDC school health programs, Department of Education, NIH, congressionally directed medical research programs via Department of Defense, etc, and through state, county, and city departments or bureaus of education, maternal and child health, corrections and juvenile justice, child and family services, and so on. *(LC1, LC5, LC6)*
	The CDC should require school health and mental health programs to use effective interventions for preventing body image disturbance and ED. *(LC5)*
	Fund research to develop, evaluate, and implement effective communications and programs to reduce mental health stigma and ED stigma among the public and health care providers. *(LC2)*
Changing context to make individuals' default decisions healthy	Add taxes on or ban or restrict sale of diet pills and other products abused for but not medically recommended for weight and shape control. *(LC5)*
	Add taxation (eg, taxes on sugar-sweetened beverages) and eliminate subsidies for highly processed foods shown to be harmful to health while subsidizing and increasing access to fresh fruits and vegetables and whole foods in neighborhoods, community programs, and schools across the spectrum of socioeconomic status through the Department of Agriculture's National School Lunch Program; ensure foods provided through

(continued on next page)

Table 1 (continued)	

Tiers of Health Impact Pyramid[25]	Examples of Public Policy Recommendations
	Departments of Education, Defense, Justice, Homeland Security, Agriculture, and so on, and state-, county-, and city-level equivalents make accessible fresh fruits and vegetables and whole foods and minimize dependence on highly processed foods shown to be harmful to health. *(LC5)*
	CMS should remove incentive payments for calculating BMI at medical visits or require primary care providers the option of opting out of weight/BMI calculation at medical visits as primary and tertiary prevention strategy. *(LC1, LC5)*
	Workplace wellness programs should be prohibited from imposing on employees incentives for weight loss or penalties for lack of weight loss. *(LC1, LC5)*
Structural interventions to change societal conditions that play a role in causing illness (eg, vastly unequal distribution of economic resources, discrimination in law and criminal justice, weight discrimination and stigma)	Ban weight and size discrimination in employment, education, public accommodations, and health care. *(LC5)* Prohibit the use of weight limits for participation in school activities (eg, sports, dance, cheerleading, etc). *(LC5)* Provide access to cafeteria environments in schools and government buildings free of weight stigmatizing messaging. *(LC5)* Update fitness standards in Department of Defense for service personnel to eliminate or modify weight standards and focus on cardiovascular health and performance. *(LC5)* Fund research into development, evaluation, and implementation of effective interventions to reduce weight-based stigma, bullying, and discrimination. *(LC5, LC6)* Reduce media images, messaging that place undue emphasis on thinness as an ideal regardless of health consequences of extreme thinness and harmful weight loss behaviors. Possible avenues to achieve this goal could include government constraints on digital manipulation of images that create false representation of size and shape, incentivizing through tax law corporate social responsibility to reduce this type of digital manipulation, and prohibiting weight discrimination in fashion/advertising modeling; incentivize corporate social responsibility to reduce weight discrimination in industry; restrict performance of cosmetic surgery on minors and advertising the procedures to minors and incentivize corporate social responsibility to avoid these types of procedures and advertising directed toward minors. *(LC5)* Ensure ED determinants considered in efforts to address food insecurity, such as through Special Supplemental Nutrition Program for Women, Infants, and Children, Supplemental Nutrition Assistance Program, and school meals programs; substance use prevention; interpersonal violence and child neglect and abuse prevention; and economic and zoning regulations that foster food swamps in low-income neighborhoods. *(LC5)* Ensure ED determinants and socioemotional health promotion considered in programs designed to address social determinants of health through support for government–community partnerships to advance health promoting environments in cities and communities (Healthy Cities public health policy innovation scorecard and funding from deBeaumont Foundation; Policies for

(continued on next page)

Table 1 (continued)	
Tiers of Health Impact Pyramid[25]	**Examples of Public Policy Recommendations**
	Action and Healthy Communities collaboratives and funding from Robert Wood Johnson Foundation; CDC's Hi-5 Interventions program, etc). *(LC5, LC6)*
	Convene and provide technical assistance and funding to support intersectoral partnerships in communities based on principles of collaborative governance to investigate complex problems presenting barriers to primary, secondary, and tertiary prevention of ED, to develop and deliberate viable solutions, and to implement and sustain effective strategies. *(LC3)*

Abbreviations: BMI, body mass index; CDC, Centers for Disease Control and Prevention; CMS, Centers for Medicare and Medicaid Services; HHS, Department of Health and Human Services; DSM-5, *Diagnostic and Statistical Manual of Mental Disorders*, 5th edition; ED, eating disorders; EPSDT, Early and Periodic Screening, Diagnosis, and Treatment; HRSA, Health Resources Services Administration; NIH, National Institutes of Health; PHQ-9, Patient Health Questionnaire-9; SAMHSA, Substance Abuse and Mental Health Services Administration; SBIRT, Screening, Brief Intervention, Referral, and Treatment; VA-CHAMPS, Civilian Health and Medical Program of the Department of Veterans Affairs.

[a] LC1-6 refer to the *Lancet* Commission report recommendation for targets to improve primary, secondary, and tertiary prevention initiatives to address global mental health crisis. See Recommendations From *Lancet* Commission on Global Mental Health for detailed explanation of *Lancet* Commission report recommendations #1 through #6.

tiers of the pyramid, for the second wave of advocacy, we substantially broaden the scope of targets to include many that are consistent with the lower 2 tiers of the Health Impact Pyramid. For instance, as shown in **Table 1**, policy advocacy initiatives consistent with the lower tiers of the pyramid could include imposing taxes on or banning the sale of diet pills and banning weight discrimination in employment, education, public accommodations, and health care.

Second-Wave Strategy 3: Establish Public Health Data Collection to Inform Policy Surveillance and Evaluation

Second-wave public policy advocacy recommendations in **Table 1** focus on interventions across the 5 tiers of the Frieden Health Impact Pyramid, but all interventions, including public policy interventions, must be informed by and monitored with surveillance and evaluation data collection activities.[30] These data are critical for government agencies to be able to use administrative tools to incentivize systems-level improvements through administrative mechanisms. It is important to note that, currently, US federal, state, and county or city public health surveillance and evaluation systems gather very little if any data related to eating disorders, disordered weight-related behaviors, or risk factors for or sequelae of eating disorders. Adding these types of eating disorders-related indicators to government public health surveillance and evaluation systems will substantially enhance efforts to determine the intended and possible unintended effects of interventions at any level.

Federal, state, and local behavioral health departments need to include eating disorders in their portfolios of process indicators (eg, the number of patients screened for an eating disorder, number of patients identified who are treated for an eating disorder, number of patients who accessed evidence-based treatment) and outcome indicators (eg, the percentage of patients with eating disorders whose symptoms stabilized within 6 months or for those whose symptoms did not stabilize, the percentage of patients who were referred to a higher level of care). These indicators need to be incorporated into existing data collection and performance improvement requirements of funded organizations, such as state hospitals, community mental health programs, and other directly funded mental health providers. These data should be incorporated into jurisdictional needs assessments and work plans, presented in annual reports, made available to researchers, and used in mental health service system planning. Because government agencies need a consistent source of data for measuring improvement on key metrics, advocates could focus on the inclusion of eating disorders and related indicators within agency, hospital, and health system clinical and quality improvement dashboards; local and state surveillance systems; and federal surveillance surveys.

Second-Wave Strategy 4: Engage Mental Health Clinicians and Researchers in Public Policy Advocacy and Collaborative Governance Initiatives

The call for clinicians and researchers to engage in public policy advocacy is not new, and participation in advocacy is already considered by many as a core requirement of ethical professional training and practice.[22,30] In fact, the imperative to engage in policy advocacy is formalized in ethical guidelines of leading professional societies. For instance, the American Psychiatric Association's "Principles of Medical Ethics with Annotations Especially Applicable to Psychiatry," states: "Psychiatrists should foster the cooperation of those legitimately concerned with the medical, psychological, social, and legal aspects of mental health and illness. Psychiatrists are encouraged to serve society by advising and consulting with the executive, legislative, and judiciary branches of the government."[31] The National Association of Social Workers' Code of Ethics makes a similarly direct call to public policy advocacy, stating, "Social workers should engage in social and political action that seeks to ensure that all people have equal access to the resources, employment, services, and opportunities they require to meet their basic human needs and to develop fully. Social workers should be aware of the impact of the political arena on practice and should advocate for changes in policy and legislation to improve social conditions to meet basic human needs and promote social justice."[32] The American Psychological Association, American Counseling Association, American Public Health Association, and other organizations similarly emphasize the ethical obligation of professional members to engage in public policy advocacy.

Both the *Lancet* Commission and Frieden underscore the importance of health research and clinical experts working in intersectoral collaborations both to address the deeply entrenched inadequacies of the global and US response to health crises and to disrupt and shift the powerful political and economic forces that impede efforts for fundamental, transformational change. They call for collaborations bringing together the public, private, and nonprofit sectors, including government, health experts, communities with lived experience, industry, and stakeholders from far beyond formal public health and health care systems. They invoke a vision of stakeholder engagement in community problem solving that could be best described as collaborative governance, although neither Frieden nor the *Lancet* Commission use this term. Collaborative governance, a concept well-developed in the public administration and management literature,[33,34] is explained by scholars Emerson and Nabatchi[33] as a way for invested stakeholders to formally work together to analyze and understand cross-cutting societal problems, particularly highly complex challenges in which no one public agency has clear, exclusive responsibility for them nor could one agency or sector reasonably be expected to solve them. They propose that collaborative governance approaches are ideal to address complex policy challenges where problems are experienced broadly across communities or society and with significant "contention between stakeholders about their interests and preferences for needs and solutions"[33(p165)]—a set of circumstances that well describes the many challenges that collectively impede progress on the primary, secondary, and tertiary prevention of eating disorders.

For mental health clinicians and researchers, there are compelling ethical reasons to consider the value of participating in collaborative governance approaches to advancing public policy to address eating disorders. The ethical values of beneficence and social justice, deeply held beliefs within many clinical professions and public health,[1,25,31,32] underscore the imperative to disrupt power imbalances that contribute to health and mental health inequities and undue burden on vulnerable communities. Leaders in public policy advocacy have cogently argued that those in more privileged positions within society—such as academic researchers, clinicians, and government public health leaders—should move toward equity, not just in the health outcomes we seek, but also in the decision making processes we engage in and support for developing policy to address the causes of inequities.[30,35] With collaborative governance initiatives, the members of communities most affected by the problems to be addressed such as individuals and family members affected by eating disorders, are equal stakeholders with mental health clinicians, researchers, and other collaborators in the process of problem definition and solution generation and implementation.[30,33,35]

In addition to the ethical reasons, the pragmatic reasons are equally compelling for mental health clinicians and researchers to join and promote collaborative governance initiatives to advance eating disorders public policy. A perception that government or the health care system or any one sector is capable of generating, implementing, and sustaining sufficiently comprehensive solutions to resolve the deep inadequacies and inequities that contribute to mental illness generally and eating disorders specifically is out of step with reality. Gradual decreases in government spending on services and programs at the federal and state levels has been ongoing for decades in the United States and have only intensified in the current era,[33,36–39] along with elimination of administrative policies that guide government agencies to take action and personnel who implement action,[40] and judicial rulings that seek to constrain government's authority to take action.[41] The combined impact of these trends is a diminished capacity of government on its own to solve complex problems.[33]

Furthermore, the types of complex mental health and social problems communities face both affect and are affected by all sectors of society and thus require engagement of all sectors to generate viable and effective policy solutions, vet and refine them against multiple stakeholder perspectives for acceptability and feasibility, and secure sustained support for implementation and enforcement over the long term.[22,30,33] Coinciding with these trends toward decreased government capacity and increasingly complex societal problems is a citizenry more technologically connected and more engaged in working with government and across sectors to generate new solutions to the challenges their communities face, unwilling to wait for problems to be solved for them or without them.[42,43] Mental health clinicians and researchers can bring much needed expertise to these collaborations, complementary to the expertise brought by the broad range of other stakeholders. In addition, because of their technical training, mental health scientists are uniquely able to ensure that empirical evidence is brought to bear in the deliberations of public policy solutions.[22] In sum, for both ethical and pragmatic reasons, identifying effective strategies and solutions to our nation's eating disorders crisis and mental health crisis more broadly requires that clinicians and researchers participate in collaborations across sectors. Although many clinicians and researchers may not have received training or accrued much experience in the methods of policy advocacy or in working in intersectoral collaborations, solving our most complex challenges in eating disorders and mental health as a whole will require this of mental health professionals. Now more than ever, graduate training programs and professional societies must include in their educational offerings training in both public policy advocacy and cross-sector collaborations to fulfill their missions and responsibilities to their members and to the communities they serve.

SUMMARY AND IMPLICATIONS

The challenges that the global mental health crisis pose to nations around the world, including to high-income nations like the United States, are coming increasingly into focus. The *Lancet* Commission on Global Mental Health's most recent report offers both a stark warning and a set of recommendations for actions nations would need to take through government platforms and public policy to address the crisis.[1] The present article focused specifically on the eating disorders crisis, and we have argued that these same *Lancet* Commission recommendations can be applied as a guide for assessing both the pertinence of goals and achievements of the first wave of eating disorders public policy advocacy over the past decade and to identify top priorities for focus in the next wave going forward. We have further argued that former CDC Director Frieden's Health Impact Pyramid offers an additional valuable tool to gauge the likely population impact of a range of possible policy advocacy initiatives under consideration.

As we have demonstrated, the first wave of US public policy advocacy for eating disorders brought national attention to the issue, made advances in mental health parity implementation, and increased federal research funding for eating disorders. The passage of the 21st Century Cures Act in 2016 marked the first time in US history that a federal law included specific provisions addressing eating disorders, an achievement made possible by concerted and coordinated advocacy by the eating disorders community. Despite these achievements in the first wave of advocacy, much work remains to be done, because still only a minority of people with eating disorders receive the specialized care that they need and substantial disparities persist by gender, race/ethnicity, body size, geographic region, and socioeconomic status in access to the primary, secondary, and tertiary prevention of eating disorders. Furthermore, many federal, state, and local policies and health care practices exacerbate eating disorders and disordered eating behaviors through either neglect or noxious effects of insufficiently evaluated programs and interventions.

Now on the cusp of the second wave of eating disorders policy advocacy in the United States, we can leverage current momentum in interest in mental health and substance use disorders globally and in the United States to further advance public policy advocacy. As we have argued, efforts must be broadened to target structural determinants of illness and inequities to maximize population impact for the primary, secondary, and tertiary prevention of eating disorders. Mental health clinicians and researchers should engage in public policy advocacy and participate in collaborative governance initiatives, ensuring the full participation of those with lived experience and a range of stakeholders across sectors. It will be essential for mental health clinicians, researchers, and the larger eating disorders community to develop a shared policy advocacy agenda and work collaboratively to maximize impact to improve population health and decrease the societal burden of eating disorders.

ACKNOWLEDGMENTS

Support for this work has been provided by the Ellen Feldberg Gordon Challenge Fund for Eating Disorders Prevention Research, Jennifer Perini Fund for Eating Disorders

Prevention Research, and Strategic Training Initiative for the Prevention of Eating Disorders. S.B. Austin is supported by training grants T71-MC-00009 and T76-MC-00001 from the Maternal and Child Health Bureau, Health Resources and Services Administration, US Department of Health and Human Services. The authors thank Millie Plotkin, Mark O'Neil, and Nicole Konstantinovica for their contributions to this article.

REFERENCES

1. Patel V, Saxena S, Lund C, et al. The Lancet Commission on global mental health and sustainable development. Lancet 2018. [Epub ahead of print].
2. Whiteford HA, Degenhardt L, Rehm J, et al. Global burden of disease attributable to mental and substance use disorders: findings from the Global Burden of Disease Study 2010. Lancet Infect Dis 2013;382(9904):1575–86.
3. Bloom DE, Cafiero ET, Jané-Llopis E, et al. The global economic burden of non-communicable diseases. Geneva (Switzerland): World Economic Forum; 2011.
4. Wang PS, Aguilar-Gaxiola S, Alonso J, et al. Use of mental health services for anxiety, mood, and substance disorders in 17 countries in the WHO world mental health surveys. Lancet 2007;370:841–50.
5. Gillum LA, Gouveia C, Dorsey ER, et al. NIH disease funding levels and burden of disease. PLoS One 2011;6(2):e16837.
6. Hudson JI, Hiripi E, Pope HG Jr, et al. The prevalence and correlates of eating disorders in the National Comorbidity Survey Replication. Biol Psychiatry 2007; 61(3):348–58.
7. LeGrange D, Swanson SA, Crow SJ, et al. Eating disorder not otherwise specified presentation in the US population. Int J Eat Disord 2012;45:711–8.
8. Smink FE, van Hoeken D, Hoek HW. Epidemiology of eating disorders: incidence, prevalence and mortality rates. Curr Psychiatry Rep 2012;14(4):406–14.
9. Franko DL, Keshaviah A, Eddy KT, et al. A longitudinal investigation of mortality in anorexia nervosa and bulimia nervosa. Am J Psychiatry 2013;170:917–25.
10. Arcelus J, Mitchell AJ, Wales J, et al. Mortality rates in patients with anorexia nervosa and other eating disorders: a meta-analysis of 36 studies. Arch Gen Psychiatry 2011;68(7):724–31.
11. Fichter MM, Quadflieg N. Mortality in eating disorders—results of a large prospective clinical longitudinal study. Int J Eat Disord 2016;49:391–401.
12. Reas DL, Williamson DA. Duration of illness predicts outcome for bulimia nervosa: a long-term follow-up study. Int J Eat Disord 2000;27(4):428–34.
13. Weissman RS, Rosselli F. Reducing the burden of suffering from eating disorders: unmet treatment needs, cost of illness, and the quest for cost-effectiveness. Behav Res Ther 2017;88:49–64.
14. Swanson SA, Crow SJ, Le Grange D, et al. Prevalence and correlates of eating disorders in adolescents. Results from the national comorbidity survey replication adolescent supplement. Arch Gen Psychiatry 2011;68(7):714–23.
15. Marques L, Alegria M, Becker AE, et al. Comparative prevalence, correlates of impairment, and service utilization for eating disorders across US ethnic groups: implications for reducing ethnic disparities in health care access for eating disorders. Int J Eat Disord 2010;44(5):412–20.
16. Becker AE, Franko DL, Speck A, et al. Ethnicity and differential access to care for eating disorder symptoms. Int J Eat Disord 2003;33:205–12.
17. Austin SB, Penfold RB, Johnson RL, et al. Clinician identification of youth abusing over-the-counter products for weight control in a large U.S. integrated health system. J Eat Disord 2013;1:40.

18. Austin SB, Ziyadeh NJ, Forman S, et al. Screening high school students for eating disorders: results of a national initiative. Preventing Chronic Disease 2008;5(4): 1–10.

19. Estimates of funding for various research, condition, and disease categories (RCDC). National Institutes of Health; 2018. Available at: https://report.nih.gov/categorical_spending.aspx. Accessed November 3, 2018.

20. Insel TR. The anatomy of NIMH funding. Bethesda (MD): National Institutes of Mental Health; 2015.

21. Gordon RS Jr. An operational classification of disease prevention. Public Health Rep 1983;98(2):107–9.

22. Tobin-Tyler E, Teitelbaum JB. Essentials of health justice: a primer. Burlington (MA): Jones & Bartlett Learning; 2018.

23. Center for Mental Health Services. 2018. Available at: https://www.samhsa.gov/about-us/who-we-are/offices-centers/cmhs. Accessed October 28, 2018.

24. National Institutes of Mental Health. Mental illness. Bethesda (MD): National Institutes of Mental Health; 2018.

25. Frieden TR. A framework for public health action: the health impact pyramid. Am J Public Health 2010;100(4):590–5.

26. Lasser KE, Himmelstein DU, Woolhandler S. Access to care, health status, and health disparities in the United States and Canada: results of a cross-national population-based survey. Am J Public Health 2006;96(7):1300–7.

27. Merikangas KR, He J-P, Burstein ME, et al. Service utilization for lifetime mental disorders in U.S. adolescents: results of the National Comorbidity Survey Adolescent Supplement (NCS-A). J Am Acad Child Adolesc Psychiatry 2011;50(1): 32–45.

28. Marmot M, Friel S, Bell R, et al, Commission on Social Determinants of Health. Closing the gap in a generation: health equity through action on the social determinant of health. Lancet 2008;372:1661–9.

29. Friel S, Bell R, Houweling TA, et al. Calling all Don Quixotes and Sancho Panzas: achieving the dream of global health equity through practical action on the social determinants of health. Glob Health Promot 2009;(Supp 1):9–13.

30. Burris S, Berman ML, Penn M, et al. The new public health law: a transdisciplinary approach to practice and advocacy. New York: Oxford University Press; 2018.

31. American Psychiatric Association. Principles of medical ethics with annotations especially applicable to psychiatry. Washington, DC: American Psychiatric Association; 2013. Available at: https://www.psychiatry.org/psychiatrists/practice/ethics. Accessed October 21, 2018.

32. National Association of Social Workers. Code of ethics. Washington, DC: National Association of Social Workers; 2018. Available at: https://www.socialworkers.org/About/Ethics/Code-of-Ethics/Code-of-Ethics-English. Accessed October 20, 2018.

33. Emerson K, Nabatchi T. Collaborative governance regimes. Washington, DC: Georgetown University Press; 2015.

34. O'Leary R, Vij N. Collaborative public management: where have we been and where are we going? Am Rev Public Adm 2012;42(5):507–22.

35. Wolff T, Minkler M, Wolfe SM, et al. Collaborating for equity and justice: moving beyond collective impact. Nonprofit Q 2016;42–53.

36. Ellwood JW, editor. Reductions in U.S. Domestic spending: how they affect state and local governments. New York: Taylor and Francis; 1982.

37. Himmelstein DU, Woolhandler S. Public health's falling share of the US health spending. Am J Public Health 2016;106(1):56–7.

38. Kaplan T. Federal budget deficit projected to soar to over $1 trillion in 2020. New York Times 2018.
39. Nabatchi T, Goerdel HT, Peffer S. Public administration in dark times: some questions for the future of the field. J Public Adm Res Theory 2011;21(s1):i29–43.
40. Lewis M. The fifth risk. New York: W.W. Norton & Company; 2018.
41. Appelbaum B. What the Hobby Lobby ruling means for America. New York Times 2014.
42. Nabatchi T, Leighniger M. Public participation for 21st Century democracy. San Francisco (CA): Jossey-Bass; 2015.
43. Fung A. Putting the public back into governance: the challenges of citizen participation and its future. Public Adm Rev 2015;75(4):1–10.

Moving?

Make sure your subscription moves with you!

To notify us of your new address, find your **Clinics Account Number** (located on your mailing label above your name), and contact customer service at:

Email: journalscustomerservice-usa@elsevier.com

800-654-2452 (subscribers in the U.S. & Canada)
314-447-8871 (subscribers outside of the U.S. & Canada)

Fax number: 314-447-8029

Elsevier Health Sciences Division
Subscription Customer Service
3251 Riverport Lane
Maryland Heights, MO 63043

*To ensure uninterrupted delivery of your subscription, please notify us at least 4 weeks in advance of move.

Printed and bound by CPI Group (UK) Ltd, Croydon, CR0 4YY

03/10/2024

01040407-0017